Assessment and Decision Making in Mental Health Nursing

Transforming Nursing Practice series

Transforming Nursing Practice is the first series of books designed to help students meet the requirements of the NMC Standards and Essential Skills Clusters for degree programmes. Each book addresses a core topic, and together they cover the generic knowledge required for all fields of practice.

Core knowledge titles:

Series editor: Professor Shirley Bach, Head of the School of Nursing and Midwifery at the University of Brighton

Personal and professional learning skills titles:

Series editors: Dr Mooi Standing, Independent Academic Consultant (UK and International) & Accredited NMC Reviewer, and Professor Shirley Bach, Head of the School of Nursing and Midwifery at the University of Brighton

You can find more information on each of these titles and our other learning resources at **www.sagepub.co.uk**. Many of these titles are also available in various e-book formats; please visit our website for more information.

Assessment and Decision Making in Mental Health Nursing

Sandra Walker, Diane Carpenter
and Yvonne Middlewick

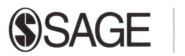 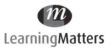

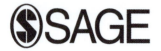 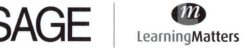

Learning Matters
An imprint of SAGE Publications Ltd
1 Oliver's Yard
55 City Road
London EC1Y 1SP

SAGE Publications Inc.
2455 Teller Road
Thousand Oaks, California 91320

SAGE Publications India Pvt Ltd
B 1/I 1 Mohan Cooperative Industrial Area
Mathura Road
New Delhi 110 044

SAGE Publications Asia-Pacific Pte Ltd
3 Church Street
#10-04 Samsung Hub
Singapore 049483

Editor: Alex Clabburn
Development editor: Caroline Sheldrick
Production controller: Chris Marke
Project manager: Diana Chambers
Marketing manager: Tamara Navaratnam
Cover design: Wendy Scott
Typeset by: Kelly Winter
Printed and bound by Henry Ling Limited, at the
Dorset Press, Dorchester, DT1 1HD

Library of Congress Control Number: 2013943599

British Library Cataloguing in Publication data

A catalogue record for this book is available from
the British Library

ISBN 0-978-1-44626-819-3
ISBN 0-978-1-44626-820-9 (pbk)

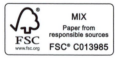

Contents

Foreword

Assessment is one of the most important aspects of mental health care yet often seems to be merely a first step in a 'production line' process – as something to 'do', perhaps even quickly get out of the way, so that the main business of caring for a person can be set in motion.

Yet full assessment of the lived experience of people with mental health challenges takes a lot of time and effort. On occasion, interpretation may have to be 'quick and dirty' under the acute demands posed by an individual's state of mind and any unfolding crisis. However, the rule should be to dwell longer on initial and continuing assessment than any other aspect of care and ensure this is achieved in a respectful, confidential and compassionate way.

For some time now, there has been concern about the way that the story of the service user is rendered in professional assessments. How closely do professionals capture the reality and experience of service users in documentation? Are such accounts accurate? Do they construct possibly misleading descriptions of a person that future practitioner-readers work from without question or challenge? Do such accounts support and advance the integrity and identity of service users? Are service users empowered or disempowered in such texts? Or are they, for example, represented as incomprehensible, manipulative or non-compliant? Writing something of the life of a service user, for that is what assessments involve, needs to be ethical and conscientious.

Assessments are biographical acts that need to be taken seriously in terms of the potential for inaccurate portrayal of service users, misdirecting decision making about them and even closing down on their futures. Care notes are written texts that endure and can be read and misread by multiple individuals in different places and at different times. At best they can helpfully guide future care. At worst, they can trap and limit the lives of our fellow human beings. Poor or incomplete assessments can lead to fatalities, poor compliance (in that what follows in decisions and care interventions might not be accurate to the person's needs and therefore refused), service user dissatisfaction (especially when their voice is ignored), poor outcomes (perhaps because key needs are missed), litigation and service user disempowerment.

Take the following case, for example, in which a GP assessed a young mother and sent a referral note stating that this mother was a prostitute who was not coping. A Community Mental Health Nurse picked up the referral and visited her at home. The flat was well maintained with plenty of toys for her young child who seemed very happy. The mother had complained to the GP that she had been feeling tired and suspected her haemoglobin might be low. But the GP had assumed she was depressed and mistook her statement that her flat had been paid for by her boyfriend as indicating a pimp–prostitute relationship. This was not the case at all and illustrates just how important it is to remain very cautious in interpreting what other people say to us and what we read about other people in referral and care notes. At all times, we should strive for accurate, shared understanding.

In healthcare settings and services there is a preference for particular kinds of stories from service users – ones that give a clear indication of the nature and progression of mental illness or symptoms that can form part of an explanatory framework. In approaching the issue of assessment it is important that we keep in mind the fragility of the information gathered and the narrative twists given by service users, relatives and practitioners.

Whenever possible, assessments should be co-constructed by the practitioner and the service user, and revisited at several points to determine whether a particular 'snapshot' on a particular day can still be considered an accurate account of the biopsychosocial status of the person or whether the information needs to be revised.

There are very real challenges, then, in interpreting people with mental health problems and how we make decisions based on assessments. Assessments will be more about story than they are about 'certainty' and 'truth', and will therefore require vigilance, our best judgements and determination to view any interpretation as potentially flawed and incomplete. Indeed, 'reading' or interpreting mental health service users requires the ability to situate and understand their stories in the contexts of many other stories or what we might even call 'life patterns'. All the time, we should remain sceptical when reading the assessments of others.

This book is a welcome reminder and resource about the core activity of assessment leading to decision making. It offers a useful introduction to these important subjects, providing ample opportunity for reflection on practice. To help the early learner, there are many nuggets of information on standards, competencies and legal/ethical matters. The scenarios bring the challenge of assessment and decision making to life and the references to other sources of information are welcome. But importantly, the book draws attention to the complexity of assessment and decision making. It avoids the trap of trying to be comprehensive in its guidance. It reminds us that assessment and decision making should always be considered provisional and met by ethical practice. Finally, it indicates that our best assessments and decision making are likely to arise from working in teams, sharing our views or insights and listening closely to the service user.

Professor Paul Crawford
Director of the Centre for Social Futures
Institute of Mental Health
The University of Nottingham

About the authors

Sandra Walker is a Senior Teaching Fellow in Mental Health at Southampton University, where she is also a doctorate student researching the patient experience of the mental health assessment in the Emergency Department. She is a Qualified Mental Health Nurse with a wide range of clinical experience spanning more than 20 years. In addition to her university work Sandra is a professional musician and does voluntary work for various mental health organisations, including being the coordinator for the Hampshire Human Library – an international initiative aimed at reducing stigmatisation through interaction and education of the public. She is the creative director of The Sanity Company, which publishes books aimed at helping children and young people to develop good mental health and problem-solving skills.

Diane Carpenter has a clinical background in Mental Health Nursing with a particular emphasis on acute care. She has taught mental health nurses and other health and social care professionals in academic and clinical environments since 1986. Her academic interests are diverse. She has a first degree in Public Sector (Health) Studies, which was primarily focused on social science broadly and public policy more specifically, and an MSc in Evidence Based Health Care from the University of Oxford – the focus of this research was suicide assessment. Her doctorate from the University of Portsmouth is in medical and social history. Diane is currently a Lecturer (Mental Health) and Programme Lead for the MSc Health Sciences.

Yvonne Middlewick has been a lecturer in the Faculty of Health Sciences at the University of Southampton since 2006, where she teaches on pre- and post-registration courses. She is a dual registered nurse (Adult and Mental Health) and much of her clinical practice has involved working with older adults with complex health needs. A key aspect of this is being able to build relationships to enable staff to work effectively with patients and their carers in a collaborative, empowering way. Yvonne believes that, although you start developing the skills to work with people early in your education, it is a continual learning and development process that continues throughout your career and is shaped by your experiences.

Acknowledgements

The authors and publisher thank Elsevier Ltd for permission to reproduce Figure 5.2, Brunswik's Lens Model, from *Clinical Decision Making and Judgement in Nursing*, C. Thompson and D. Dowding, Churchill Livingstone 2002 (p. 87).

The authors and publisher also wish to thank the reviewers of early drafts of this book for their helpful advice.

Introduction

Who is this book for?

This book is written for student nurses currently undertaking their qualifications. It will also be useful for junior nurses who are just beginning their careers and anyone who has to regularly conduct mental health assessments.

Why *Assessment and Decision Making in Mental Health Nursing*?

Assessment is a core function of mental health nursing and as such a core learning requirement for pre-registration nurses. Assessment is the means by which patients' needs are ascertained and appropriate treatment plans created in conjunction with the patient. Getting assessment right is essential for student nurses in order for them to become effective practitioners. It is taught from the beginning of the undergraduate curriculum with a focus on skills from the end of the first year onwards; however, the student nurse will encounter assessment in practice from the very first placement. This book aims to provide useful practical tools to aid the student nurse in developing good assessment and decision-making practice.

Book structure

Chapter 1 introduces you to the principles, practicalities and purpose of a mental health (MH) assessment. We begin an exploration of assumptions and preconceived ideas about other people and how these impact on the assessment process. The reasons for assessment are considered and theory is related directly to practice through activities and case studies. The chapter first looks at assessment in general terms, then the assessment as part of the mental health nursing process along with the purpose of assessment in mental health settings. Also considered are the practical aspects of carrying out an assessment, looking at when and why assessment may occur in mental health.

In Chapter 2 we concentrate on engagement, considering how to build relationships with the people involved with the assessment process generally within the context of mental health practice. We also consider how nurses can build rapport with people using their services, thereby enabling them to engage in the assessment process and begin their recovery journey. Borne in mind throughout this chapter are the four requests from service users, which are in line with what recent reports and policies are telling us: to listen to service users, to treat them with compassion, to treat them as equals and to continue to strive on their behalf.

Chapter 3 invites a more critical consideration of assessment, developing some of the ideas and building on the reflective practice opportunities of the previous chapters. This chapter offers the opportunity to consider critically whether or not to read service users' notes before assessing them. It considers the merits of comprehensive history taking and identifying a history-taking structure and discusses the relative merits of universal/holistic online and bespoke condition-specific assessments. There is critical debate about the issues associated with involving service users meaningfully in their assessments, as, while drawing the reader's attention to a range of assessment tools, it is important to remember that the therapeutic relationship and engagement with service users and carers is paramount and that the practitioner is more than the sum of his or her toolkit.

The purpose of Chapter 4 is to consider some of the problems encountered in carrying out assessments in mental health nursing and exploring some potential solutions. This chapter revisits some of the political, technical and legal issues encountered in Chapter 1, then looks in more detail at the economic issues that can challenge assessment. The social and cultural impact of assessment is considered too, with a closer look at how stigmatisation can affect self-perception and the intricacies of involving family and carers in the assessment process. The chapter then moves on to consider some of the ethical issues that can become a challenge in the assessment process and includes a further look at practical challenges such as talking to people who are highly emotional. This chapter ends by considering some of the risk issues that may pose a challenge to assessment.

The assessment process leads quite naturally on to decision making and in Chapter 5 the basic principles of decision making are considered and explored along with the complexity of the process via text and exercises. Some of the theory on decision making and how it applies to mental health practice is covered, with a focus on certain models that can be useful in decision making and how practitioners can learn from them. The importance of clinical judgement is also explored and the essential element of service user involvement. At the end of the chapter, risk in decision making, in particular the principle of positive risk taking, is considered.

Following on from previous chapters, Chapter 6 continues to consider the importance of engaging the patient and carers in the assessment process to ensure an accurate picture of the patient's issues. In this chapter different outcomes that may result from assessment are discussed along with the complex nature of sharing information and some of the ethical dilemmas this can present.

In the final chapter, some of the important things to consider after the assessment are discussed. It includes a look at what might happen when things go wrong, assessments don't work out as hoped and consideration of referring on after the assessment. The most important points to consider in looking after yourself in the assessment process are covered in this chapter. The complexities of assessment are clearly demonstrated, as well as the different outcomes that can be the result, while considering some of the legal and ethical implications of assessment. This chapter also reflects on the outcomes of assessment when using an evidenced-based approach compared to a locally adapted assessment and considers some of the difficulties inherent in the complex healthcare systems we are currently operating in.

Requirements for the NMC *Standards for Pre-registration Nursing Education* and the Essential Skills Clusters

The Nursing and Midwifery Council (NMC) has established standards of competence to be met by applicants to different parts of the register, and these are the standards it considers necessary for safe and effective practice. In addition to the competencies, the NMC has set out specific skills that nursing students must be able to perform at various points of an education programme. These are known as Essential Skills Clusters (ESCs). This book is structured so that it will help you to understand and meet the competencies and ESCs required for entry to the NMC register. The relevant competencies and ESCs are presented at the start of each chapter so that you can clearly see which ones the chapter addresses. There are *generic standards* that all nursing students irrespective of their field must achieve, and *field-specific standards* relating to each field of nursing, that is, mental health, children's, learning disability and adult nursing.

This book includes the latest standards for 2010 onwards, taken from *Standards for Pre-registration Nursing Education* (NMC, 2010b). For links to the pre-2010 standards, please visit the website for the book at www.learningmatters.co.uk/nursing.

Learning features

Activities

Throughout the book you will find activities in the text that will help you to make sense of, and learn about, the material being presented by the authors.

Some activities ask you to reflect on aspects of practice, or your experience of it, or the people or situations you encounter. *Reflection* is an essential skill in nursing, and it helps you to understand the world around you and often to identify how things might be improved. Other activities will help you develop key skills such as your ability to *think critically* about a topic in order to challenge received wisdom, or your ability to *research a topic and find appropriate information and evidence*, and to be able to *make decisions* using that evidence in situations that are often difficult and time-pressured. Finally, communication and working as part of a team are core to all nursing practice, and some activities will ask you to carry out *group activities* or think about your *communication skills* to help develop these.

All the activities require you to take a break from reading the text, think through the issues presented and carry out some independent study, possibly using the internet. Where appropriate, there are sample answers presented at the end of each chapter, and these will help you to understand more fully your own reflections and independent study. Remember, academic study will always require independent work; attending lectures will never be enough to be successful on your programme, and these activities will help to deepen your knowledge and understanding of the issues under scrutiny and give you practice at working on your own.

You might want to think about completing these activities as part of your personal development plan (PDP) or portfolio. After completing the activity, write it up in your PDP or portfolio in a section devoted to that particular skill, then look back over time to see how well you are developing. You can also do more of the activities for a key skill that you have identified a weakness in, which will help build your skill and confidence in this area.

Case studies and scenarios

The case studies and scenarios in this book have been carefully chosen to aid your development and help you to think critically about policy and practice. They are often quite complex and, in this way, provide a useful and realistic arena for you to explore, test out your decisions and make mistakes in a safe environment while then providing you with the opportunity to learn from them. The activities overall will allow you to practise some key skills and help you to develop a useful toolkit of techniques that you can access when you need them, enabling you to develop solid, ethical and high-quality practice at the beginning of your nursing career.

Chapter 1
Introduction to assessment principles

Sandra Walker and Diane Carpenter

NMC Standards for Pre-registration Nursing Education

This chapter will address the following competencies:

Domain 1: Professional values

5. All nurses must fully understand the nurse's various roles, responsibilities and functions, and adapt their practice to meet the changing needs of people, groups, communities and populations.

Domain 2: Communication and interpersonal skills

1. All nurses must build partnerships and therapeutic relationships through safe, effective and non-discriminatory communication. They must take account of individual differences, capabilities and needs.

Domain 3: Nursing practice and decision-making

3. All nurses must carry out comprehensive, systematic nursing assessments that take account of relevant physical, social, cultural, psychological, spiritual, genetic and environmental factors, in partnership with service users and others through interaction, observation and measurement.

3.1 **Mental health nurses** must be able to apply their knowledge and skills in a range of evidence-based individual and group psychological and psychosocial interventions, to carry out systematic needs assessments, develop case formulations and negotiate goals.

NMC Essential Skills Clusters

This chapter will address the following ESCs:

Cluster: Organisational aspects of care

9. People can trust the newly registered graduate nurse to treat them as partners and work with them to make a holistic and systematic assessment of their needs; to develop a personalised plan that is based on mutual understanding and respect for

continued . . .

their individual situation promoting health and well-being, minimising risk of harm and promoting their safety at all times.

By entry to the register:

12.   In partnership with the person, their carers and their families, makes a holistic, person centred and systematic assessment of physical, emotional, psychological, social, cultural and spiritual needs, including risk, and together, develops a comprehensive personalised plan of nursing care.

Chapter aims

By the end of this chapter you should be able to:

*   define assessment in mental health nursing;
*   begin to understand the process of assessment in mental health nursing;
*   begin to demonstrate an awareness of your own preconceptions and how these might impact on the assessment process;
*   list basic principles that apply to the assessment process;
*   understand the purpose of assessment in mental health practice.

Introduction

Case study

Barbara is a 60-year-old woman who was admitted to an emergency department following a large paracetamol overdose. A practitioner from the resident mental health liaison team carried out a mental health assessment once it was clear that Barbara was in no physical danger from her overdose.

The practitioner took Barbara to a private room and asked questions about the situation that had led to the overdose, the intention of her actions, her mental state, and her social situation and risk. During the assessment Barbara showed no signs of mental ill health and described no symptoms. She explained that she had a new job where her boss had expected her to take a computing exam that terrified her and that, rather than talking to her boss, she took the overdose. She regretted what she had done and no longer felt suicidal.

The assessment took about 45 minutes and the practitioner and Barbara worked together to make an action plan so that Barbara could address the issues that had led to the overdose in the first place. These included practising being more assertive so that she could explain the situation to her boss should it recur. Barbara did not require any formal follow-up from mental health services but her GP was informed.

The mental health (MH) assessment is a very important aspect of mental healthcare. It is essential in allowing us, as healthcare providers, to find out what people need. Care plans, treatment delivery and services are all based around patient need, and assessment is one of the primary ways we have to help us decide what people need. Getting this process right is extremely important and learning to carry out assessments is something you will need to do as mental health student nurses. If the practitioner had not assessed Barbara in the case study above, the outcome could have been very different; perhaps assumptions may have been made regarding her risk, which could have led to her being admitted to a psychiatric unit for further assessment and which would have been a costly and unnecessary course of action, as well as distressing for Barbara.

The purpose of this chapter is to introduce you to the principles, practicalities and purpose of an MH assessment. You will begin to explore your own assumptions and preconceived ideas about other people and how these impact on the assessment process. The reasons for assessment will become clear and you will be able to relate the theory directly to your practice through the activities and case studies.

The chapter will first look at assessment in general terms, then at assessment as part of the mental health nursing process along with the purpose of assessment in mental health settings. We will consider the practical aspects of carrying out an assessment, look at when and why we might assess and think about informal and formal assessment in mental health.

What is assessment and how does it fit in the nursing process?

On a day-to-day basis we regularly assess for risks, opportunities and gains. We look both ways before crossing the road and assess the speed of oncoming traffic, weighing up the likelihood of being knocked down if we step into the road, before deciding to cross; we assess the likelihood of a positive response before asking someone out on a date; we assess the likelihood of food poisoning before ordering fish from the menu; we assess the likelihood of someone bursting into tears before asking them if they feel OK. In all these cases we consider past experiences, the current situation, the history of the case and available information, and then predict outcomes before deciding on the action most likely to lead to the desired outcome. These 'assessments' may take place in a split second, perhaps without our being aware that we are actually undertaking such a process at all.

When we make an assessment in mental health nursing, however, it requires a conscious and deliberate approach. So it is helpful to consider what assessment actually means, especially within mental health nursing.

Activity 1.1   *Reflection*

- Spend a few minutes thinking about what assessment means for you.
- Write a short definition.

Consider your answers in light of the discussion below.

The Penguin English Dictionary defines 'assessment' as:

1. *Determine the rate or amount of.*
2. *To make an official valuation of.*
3. *To estimate the quality or worth of, to evaluate.*

Oxford Dictionaries Online define 'assessment' as *the action of assessing someone or something* and 'assess' as:

1. *Evaluate or estimate the nature, ability or quality of.*
2. *Calculate or estimate the price or value of.*
3. *Set the value of a tax, fine etc. for (a person or property) at a specified level.*

How closely does this match your definition of assessment in Activity 1.1; and how does this compare to assessment in mental health nursing?

Barker (2004) defines assessment as:

> *The decision-making process, based upon the collection of relevant information, using a formal set of ethical criteria, that contributes to an overall estimation of a person and his circumstances.*

Activity 1.2   *Critical thinking*

- Consider the above definitions and apply them to Barbara in the first case study. Note down any conflicts you might see.

Consider your answer in light of the discussion below. An outline answer is also provided at the end of the chapter.

The practitioner assessing Barbara would have asked questions to find out if she had been suicidal and if she still had any suicidal intent. From the answer to these questions the practitioner would have been able to estimate the risk of Barbara taking another overdose. Other questions, looking at the social situation for example, would help the practitioner decide if Barbara had enough support at home to help her should the situation that led to the overdose happen again. So, *estimation of risk* is certainly one way that the definitions all fit; however, when considering the value of something as in the first two definitions, how well does this fit with Barker's definition of contributing to an 'overall estimation of a person'? Here we are in murkier waters, as the practitioner's values will have a direct influence on this estimation and could lead to decisions based on the sort of person Barbara is perceived to be rather than on the person Barbara believes she is. Are we setting the value or worth of a person when we assess them? We will explore this further in Chapters 2 and 4.

For the purposes of this book we define assessment in mental health nursing as:

> *A process by which we ascertain the history, current situation and potential treatment of a person requesting/requiring healthcare.*

This fits nicely with Barker's definition above. Barker (2004) maintains that the actual term 'assessment' has come to have something to do with estimating the character of something or someone. He states that, in nursing, the assessment may seek an answer to the question – 'What does it mean to be this person?'

Within the medical model framework an assessment may aim to find out what is *medically* wrong with the person. It focuses on signs and symptoms usually elicited by taking a medical history and by physical examination. This process will usually lead to a diagnosis (Aggleton and Chalmers, 2000). In nursing, we aim to get a total picture of the patient (not just their illness) and how he or she can be helped in terms of moving towards individual goals, which do not always include cure. This requires data about patient, family, social, emotional and environmental factors, malfunctions in coping for that individual, coping abilities, and strengths and risk factors. These factors then create a psychosocial picture that, when complemented by the medical model, gives us a comprehensive bio-psychosocial overview of the position of the patient, how they got to where they are and clues about how to help them to move forward to a more healthy place or a desired outcome.

Mental health nursing is an important profession that combines an artistic use of self with the science of medical, psychological and social research evidence and theory. Mental health nurses provide holistic, patient-centred care in a variety of settings across healthcare (ISPN, 2006) and assessment is the tool that we use, in all its various forms, to help decide with patients which avenues of care/courses of action are the best ones for them as individuals.

Informal and formal assessment

All healthcare trusts have preferred formal assessment tools that they use, for example, on admission, in mental state examination, in risk assessments, and so on. Some of these assessments are nationally recommended, but some may also be developed locally according to the needs of the service.

Activity 1.3   *Critical thinking*

Find an example of a formal assessment tool used in your clinical area. Read it and consider the following in light of your current clinical area:

- What practical issues would arise in carrying out this assessment?
- How easy would it be to carry out this assessment?
- Would any personal issues arise for you in carrying out this assessment?

As this activity is based on your own choice of tool, there is no outline answer at the end of the chapter.

There are many opportunities for informal assessment as a mental health nurse. As a skilled practitioner you will be assessing a patient each time you talk to him or her. In order to notice significant changes, however small, you need to know your patient. Every interaction is an opportunity. A game of pool, for example, can give you invaluable information about your patient's mental state; one-to-one observation is the ideal time to connect with your patient and discover more about the person and what makes him or her tick.

Case study

Gemma, a mental health nurse, used to work on a low-secure unit that provided care for patients who had severe and enduring mental health problems with associated criminal convictions. She often did one-to-one observations of a young man with paranoid schizophrenia. He was not one for chatting, but in the course of her observations Gemma noticed that he paced the room repeatedly, becoming more and more agitated when the resident in the next room played his music loudly. Although he did not offer any information when Gemma asked him, she asked the neighbour to turn down his music and stop playing it so loudly. In a very short time Gemma could see that the young man concerned had calmed and was able to tell her that the music was overstimulating and, combined with his auditory hallucinations, was causing him to become agitated.

Here, Gemma had correctly assessed the situation and taken action that resulted in an improvement for that patient.

The purpose of assessment

What is the purpose of assessment in mental health nursing and what are our aims? The main reasons for carrying out an MH assessment are:

- to identify mental disorder;
- to identify psychological or other problems;
- to identify if further support or care is required;
- to identify risks;
- to learn more about the person in order to create an appropriate action plan with them.

In order to discover these things we need to build a relationship with the person, and we will look more closely at this in Chapter 2.

There are many other reasons for carrying out an assessment in mental healthcare: you may be asked to assess someone's mental state prior to them going on community leave; an assessment may be carried out to ascertain if a person requires inpatient or outpatient care; you may be asked to assess over time to make a judgement as to whether a patient's treatment is effective; there may be a conflict of need between two patients and you may be asked to assess them and help decide which patient gets the resource. You will become more familiar with many of the different assessment types throughout the course of this book.

Consider the person in the following case study.

> **Case study**
>
> *Lucy is a 20-year-old woman. She is tall, blonde and of slight build. She is cleanly presented, well made up and smartly dressed in a white shirt and short black skirt. She has a black eye and has come to the GP with low mood and lethargy. The GP is concerned about her and asks the practice mental health nurse, Gemma, to assess Lucy.*

Write down your initial thoughts about Lucy, and do not censor them. Put them to one side as we will come back to them later.

Let us initially consider the possible aims in carrying out an assessment of Lucy. These could be:

- assessment of her mental state – looking for signs and/or symptoms of depression;
- looking for triggers for her current mood;
- discovering if she has any pertinent history;
- deciding what treatment, if any, would be appropriate;
- looking for problems affecting her quality of life;
- reduction of risks.

Hildegarde Peplau (1988) states that:

> *Every nurse in all nursing situations uses three principal operations: observation, interpretation and intervention. What is observed or noticed must be interpreted; that is, the raw data must be transformed into some meaningful explanation.*

In the case of Lucy, above, the nurse would be observing her behaviour; asking questions about her history and current situation; listening to the story, as told from Lucy's perspective; and interpreting all this information and considering which interventions may be most effective in helping Lucy decide what options are available in terms of treatment and next steps.

The assessment we initiate will be affected by our own values and judgements. It is essential that we are aware of these when entering into an assessment situation. So, in the case of Lucy, Gemma (the mental health nurse) suspects that Lucy has been the victim of domestic violence due to her black eye, but were she only to ask questions to gather information to prove her theory she could miss a lot of other very important information and interpret what Lucy says in light of the belief that she holds.

Assessment practicalities

There are many practical aspects to consider when undertaking an MH assessment. These include privacy, confidentiality, note taking and resources, which we will look at now in more detail. You will have undergone some form of health assessment during your life. Spend some time reliving one of these in the following reflection.

Think back to a time when you have been interviewed in a healthcare setting as a patient.

- What made you feel comfortable?
- What made you feel uncomfortable?

Consider your answers in light of the discussion below.

There are some very simple things that can make us feel uncomfortable when we are being assessed, such as lack of eye contact (e.g. looking at the computer monitor instead of you) or too much eye contact, or the assessor continually clock-watching, not allowing you to finish your sentences when you are telling him or her what is wrong, and getting your name wrong – these are some of the common ones. So how can we ensure that people are comfortable when we are asking them to share the very personal information we need in order to complete an MH assessment?

NICE guidance

The National Institute for Health and Clinical (now Care) Excellence (NICE, 2011) published some guidance on improving the service user experience in mental health services, which suggests some important considerations when carrying out an assessment:

- *ensure there is enough time for the service user to describe and discuss their problems;*
- *allow enough time towards the end of the appointment for summarising the conclusions of the assessment and for discussion, with questions and answers;*
- *explain the use and meaning of any clinical terms used;*
- *explain and give written material in an accessible format about any diagnosis given;*
- *give information about different treatment options, including drug and psychological treatments, and their side effects, to promote discussion and shared understanding;*
- *offer support after the assessment, particularly if sensitive issues, such as childhood trauma, have been discussed.*

(1.3.3)

✳ Privacy

Case study

Jim has taken an overdose of painkillers. He has been treated and is no longer in physical danger. The mental health practitioner assesses him at his bedside in the four-bedded ward where the bed spaces are separated by curtains.

Privacy is an obvious requirement for any kind of assessment. Yet the Department of Health consistently refers to it in its guidance documents showing that it is not always considered automatically in healthcare (see NHS Executive, 2000, as an example). For an MH assessment privacy is extremely important. It should be carried out somewhere where the patient can speak freely without fear of being overheard. In practice this principle can be very difficult to facilitate, as in Jim's case above. When the unit is busy, demand for private rooms is high and space is at a premium. If you have to carry out an assessment in unfavourable conditions, explain the problem to the patient and encourage him or her to speak as quietly as possible. It can also help to ensure that you have pen and paper to hand to allow the patient to write down particularly sensitive issues, though of course this is not an option for everyone.

Confidentiality

At the outset of any MH assessment it is important to outline your boundaries to the patient on the subject of confidentiality. It is not always possible to maintain full confidentiality and the patient needs to be aware of this from the beginning. All nurses are bound by strict rules around confidentiality and these are clearly outlined in the NMC *Code* (2008a).

NMC guidelines for confidentiality

The Code: Standards of conduct, performance and ethics for nurses and midwives (2008a) makes the following statements.

- *You must respect people's right to confidentiality.*
- *You must ensure people are informed about how and why information is shared by those who will be providing their care.*
- *You must disclose information if you believe someone may be at risk of harm, in line with the law of the country in which you are practising.*

(p3)

Consider the following activity.

Activity 1.5   *Decision making*

Imagine you are nursing Jim, from the case study on page 12, and he starts to tell you 'something important' and asks you to promise not to tell anyone else.

- If you were the nurse, what would you say to Jim?
- Under what circumstances would you have to tell someone else?

Outline answers are provided at the end of the chapter.

When a friend says they want to share a secret with us we may huddle up and look forward to a shared confidence; but in practising as a nurse it is very important to remember the demands of professional conduct. In this instance, when Jim asks to share it is essential that you ensure that he is aware that, depending on the nature of his secret, you may not be able to keep it confidential. You can go on to state that the reasons for this could be if he was indicating that someone may be at risk, particularly a child, or if he revealed that he had intentions of harming himself or others. In this way Jim is given the power to decide whether or not he wants to go on and share his story, knowing the boundaries required of you as a professional.

Note taking during assessment

Should you take notes during an assessment, or not? There is no clear right or wrong and it will often come down to personal or patient choice. Different establishments may provide guidance about this, but increasingly, in light of the amount of time MH assessments take, it is expected that notes will be taken at the time, with the understanding that it is not always considered ideal from the patient's perspective. Some nurses prefer to take notes if they are concerned about remembering everything important, and explain this at the beginning of any assessment. Some nurses never take notes at the time, but once the assessment is complete immediately write it up. You will find the way that works best for you in your clinical environment. If you choose, or are expected, to write notes during the assessment it is essential that you explain to the patient what you are doing and why, and how the notes will be used (e.g. deal with issues of data protection and confidentiality). If you choose to write notes after the assessment, do not wait too long to do it, as the longer the time passes, the more you will forget.

Resources available to the service user

As a practitioner you need to become aware of the resources you have to refer people on to if required, to ensure that any offer of follow-up is realistic and deliverable.

Case study

Graham is a 24-year-old man who attended the emergency department following a fight and was referred to the mental health team for an assessment as he expressed some suicidal thoughts to the suture nurse. During his assessment it became clear that he was having a serious problem with anger management, which was endangering his relationship with his girlfriend. He did not want to lose this relationship as she was 'the best thing in his life' and he felt he needed anger management counselling. A full MH assessment indicated that there were no other signs or symptoms of mental illness and he therefore did not meet the criteria for further support from mental health services, which would have included anger management. There were no other locally available avenues for anger management work; therefore, the only option was private counselling, which he could not afford. Graham had made it clear during assessment that he was not actively suicidal and had been expressing frustration to the nurse rather than meaning to suggest actual harm to himself. Despite the clear need, the nurse had to discharge Graham back to the care of his GP with no further follow-up.

If the nurse stated at the outset that it was not clear whether there was any anger management service available locally, but that he or she would check, Graham would not have his hopes raised unnecessarily. A knowledge of the local resources available is very helpful in this sort of scenario, and ensuring we do not promise something that does not exist is very important.

A full MH assessment takes time to carry out; it is important that you ensure, as far as is possible, a realistic amount of time to cover the ground required. The policy implementation guides for Mental Health Liaison Services (Aitken, 2007), a service that carries out many MH assessments, suggest that the average time for a face-to-face assessment is 90 minutes.

Your impact on the assessment process

We are human beings first and foremost, and therefore we are also subject to prejudices and values that can be at odds with those of our patients. It is very important that we are aware of these prejudices and know ourselves well so that our values can be kept separate from those of our patients. In the following case study, activity and discussion we explore this further.

Case study

Greg is 34, lives alone in a bedsit and is being supported by the crisis team through a particularly difficult bereavement. He is visited by Julie, a nurse working in the crisis team, who is to assess him for discharge. He is unwashed, his bedsit is a mess and there are many empty beer cans lying around. Julie can't stand the smell and keeps wrinkling her nose up, which Greg notices. She believes that Greg is still very low as he clearly has not been looking after himself or his environment and it appears he may be drinking heavily too. When she asks Greg how he feels, he states that he thinks he is a lot better and feels able to carry on without any further support. Julie does not believe this and tries to convince Greg that he needs the team to continue to monitor him.

Activity 1.6	*Critical thinking*

- What are the values that Julie is exhibiting here?
- What assumptions have you made from this case study and what do they say about your values?
- What should Julie be asking Greg?
- How do you think Greg will be feeling about being persuaded to stay with the team when he feels he is ready to be discharged?

Outline answers are provided at the end of the chapter.

Julie clearly believes that healthy people are clean and tidy; this is one of her values and if she had allowed herself or her home environment to get that dirty and smelly it would indeed be an indicator of serious depression. However, in Greg's case this may not be so. The nurse must ask Greg what state his bedsit is normally in and how often he feels it is necessary to wash, and she must ascertain why the beer cans are lying about – the team should already have information about how much alcohol Greg normally drinks. If it is quite normal for Greg to smell and for his bedsit to be a mess, this would not indicate a problem at all. Are the beer cans there because Greg has had friends round the night before and they were watching the football? This could indicate that he is much better as he is socialising and not that he has a burgeoning alcohol problem. Greg could be feeling very undermined by the nurse's insistence that he needs continued support. He may doubt himself, which could have longer-term impact on his belief in how well he can manage his problems. He could also be insulted by the nurse continually wrinkling her nose in disgust.

You could ask yourself the following questions before carrying out any MH assessment and then use them to guide your process of enquiry.

- Why am I carrying out this assessment?
- What is the aim of this assessment?
- When would be the best time to assess?
- How will I gather the information I need?
- How will I decide what this information means?
- Might the person function differently under other conditions?
  (Adapted from Barker, 2004)

One of the most common complaints is that a patient has to go through repeated assessments and, if the assessment is being carried out for the benefit of the system and will not move the care of the patient forward, it may be unethical to carry it out. Clear aims are essential in ensuring that both the nurse and the patient have expectations that can be met by the process of assessment. If the patient fears admission to hospital, he or she may not share information honestly with you; however, if you are able to clearly state that you are going to make every effort to help the person remain in the community to receive necessary care, he or she may be able to relax and be more honest. Sometimes assessments are requested, in emergency care for example, at unreasonable times of the day or night and it can be difficult to negotiate a more reasonable time. When this happens it is important to remember that the well-being of the patient is paramount and a different time should be negotiated wherever possible.

Looking for a connection

The appearance and performance of things are not always related – the colour of a car will not impact on the performance of its engine. We are often required to look for similar connections in the people we are assessing. We might collect information about the appearance of the person (presentation) and how he or she behaves (performance) and then see if we can understand the person better by combining these two viewpoints and making connections. Remember Lucy from the case study (page 11), whose presentation included a black eye, low mood and lethargy? Did the notes you made after reading the case study include presentation or performance? Her appearance led Gemma, the mental health nurse, to suspect that Lucy was the victim of domestic violence and that this may be causing depression, hence the low mood and lethargy. However, on closer questioning it turned out that Lucy had been hit in the face with a tennis ball during a game with a friend. So Gemma revised her theory about the depression because of this new information about Lucy's performance and continued to ask questions to explore the possible reasons for the low mood and lethargy.

Again, it is clear that being aware of our own values and preconceptions is essential in making sure we do not make dangerous assumptions in the assessment process.

Assessment principles

All assessments share the same principles.

- A reliable decision can only be made if reliable information is available.
- By studying people carefully, methodically and with the minimum of bias we are more likely to be able to reliably help them.

There is a difference between a nursing assessment and judgements we might make about the weather, cars or objects. Your professional assessment may be of crucial importance; in some cases it might make the difference between life and death. Assessment involves looking at the person with a view to gaining a picture that will help us to see him or her as a unique human being.

> ## Case study
>
> *Brenda has mild dementia, lives alone and attends a local memory clinic twice a week. She has a dosset box in order to help her manage her medication. She brings the dosset box with her to the clinic so that the nurses can assess how she is managing. Brenda tells the nurse that she is concerned that she can't always remember what day it is and whether or not she has taken the tablets, but the dosset box looks like it has been used correctly with the time and date corresponding with the current day. The nurse prefers to believe the evidence of her eyes and not the report of a lady with mild dementia, reassures Brenda that she is doing really well and sends her home with her next dosset box intact.*
>
> *Two days later Brenda is in hospital as she has been found wandering the streets in a confused and semiconscious state having taken an accidental overdose of her medication.*

In this case the nurse believed that she was a more reliable source of information than Brenda, and therefore took no action on Brenda's concerns, which resulted in a nearly catastrophic situation.

In the remainder of this section we will look at the important political, economic, social, technical and legal aspects of assessment.

Political aspects of assessment

Assessments have to take place in accordance with local and national policies and guidelines, for example the National Service Frameworks (NSFs) and the NICE guidelines. In the area you work there will be policies designed to support the practice of assessment and following these policies ensures that you are following best practice and will be supported by your employer should things go wrong.

Activity 1.7   *Evidence-based practice and research*

Find a clinical guideline from NICE (www.nice.org.uk) that corresponds to a clinical area you work in and see what the recommendations are for assessment in that area.

As this activity concerns your own clinical area, there is no outline answer at the end of the chapter.

Economic issues in assessment

Patients have repeatedly complained about being asked the same question time and time again by different practitioners. Apart from distressing the patient, this becomes an expensive exercise in terms of practitioner time. Ask your patients if they have been assessed, how long ago and by whom. Are there recent notes from a previous assessment you could use as a starting point to check the details, rather than asking the same questions again?

There is also the danger of 'false positives' (seeing a risk when there isn't one). Very risk-averse assessments can result in unnecessary care and treatment that can carry a very high cost for both the service and the patient. Talking the situation through with colleagues is a good way of ensuring that you are not being overcautious and restricting the patient's recovery.

Case study

Rob has a diagnosis of borderline personality disorder and has a comprehensive care plan, created in collaboration with him, that covers what the crisis team should do if he contacts the team making threats to harm himself. He and his whole care team agreed that admission was counterproductive for him and generally made him feel worse rather than better. They developed a set of clear guidelines regarding personal responsibility, supportive phone calls and visits in order to avoid admission in the future.

Rob phoned the crisis team in the middle of the night as he had thoughts of self-harm and he was asked to come in to be assessed. The practitioner assessing him was unwilling to take a positive risk by following the care package and admitted him to the acute ward. Rob felt he was a failure for being admitted and his wider team were angry that his care package had been ignored, resulting in an expensive admission that could have been avoided.

There is also a risk of 'false negatives' (seeing no risk where one clearly exists) in assessment. If a patient's needs are not understood and acted upon, the resulting lack of required care could lead to catastrophic events that will be very expensive and time consuming to investigate. Compensation for avoidable errors is a large part of NHS budgets. Question carefully, and avoid making assumptions, to minimise the risk of this occurring.

Case study

Ruth had been admitted to the acute ward with severe depression following the death of her newborn baby. She had been on the ward for three days and was a model patient. She was assessed for home treatment and said she would rather be at home where her baby's things were. Rather than consider this as a potential risk it was seen as a request to go home and she was discharged to the care of the home treatment team. The same evening she was admitted to intensive care at the local district hospital following a serious overdose.

In the case study above, Ruth was not asked about feelings of low mood or suicide; her outward appearance and behaviour were taken as being representative of her internal world. Research shows that people are at highest risk of self-harm in the seven days following discharge and there is also evidence that a number of people who have decided they are going to end their lives present a happier face to the world just prior to acting on their suicidal thoughts. In the light of this, staff on the ward were remiss in making assumptions about how she was actually feeling. Ruth gave a clue when she said she would rather be at home where her baby's things were – a question here about suicidal thoughts may have unearthed her plans.

As nurses, when we identify a need as practitioners, we have a duty to provide treatment and care wherever possible, while at the same time being realistic about resources available and honest with the patient about what we can offer. It is better not to make promises in the first place than to have to break them later. Remember that we discovered this in the case study about Graham on page 14?

Social issues in assessment

When a person undertakes an MH assessment it may identify problems that will impact on that person's view of themselves in society. It may change the way his or her friends and family associate with the person, and it can even affect his or her work status and financial stability. You need to be aware of these important issues when undertaking an assessment or acting as an advocate for a patient being assessed.

Activity 1.8   *Reflection*

The Time to Change website (http://time-to-change.org.uk) has many videos from people with mental health issues who have had life-changing experiences regarding their social circumstances following assessment and diagnosis.

- Go on to the website and watch some of these short films.
- After watching some of the films write a brief reflection regarding the social issues that each person has had to deal with. Imagine you were diagnosed with a mental illness, for example depression, and consider how your own life would be affected: Who would you tell? Who would you avoid telling and why?

As this activity is based on your own reflection, there is no outline answer at the end of the chapter.

It is very important to be aware of the social impact that may occur as a result of assessment. Talking to the family, with the patient's permission, about the presenting problem may help diffuse some of their concerns and prejudices around mental illness. It is equally important to avoid the careless use of labels; for example, describing behaviour as 'borderline' to a colleague can convey an unjustified label for the patient that could be hard to shake off, even though the person may not have been diagnosed with borderline personality disorder.

Technical issues in assessment

Increasingly, clinical areas are using computer-based notes, records and assessments that require the relevant technological skills for inputting data and also knowledge of the legal framework for data protection. Most employers now expect at least basic levels of computer literacy. Data protection training is generally offered at a local level, but you have a responsibility to make sure you are fully aware of the data protection requirements for your area. More information on data protection can be found on the Department of Health website (see 'Useful websites' below).

Some assessments may also require the use of technology, for example testing blood glucose levels. If the glucometer is not calibrated properly, or the patient has not washed his or her hands since handling fruit, the result may be incorrect. This could seriously affect the assessment we perform. Training should be offered by your clinical area in using these technical facilities.

Legal issues in assessment

As we have already seen, nurses have a duty of care, which is a legally binding expectation of healthcare practitioners. It describes the obligations implicit in your role as a health or social care worker (NMC, 2008a).

Failure to make an assessment when required to do so by local or national guidance, or making inaccurate assessments, may be grounds for claims of negligence. Negligence is defined as harm resulting to a patient as a result of carelessness on the part of the nurse (Griffith and Tengnah, 2010). You must have knowledge of local and national policies regarding assessment for your clinical area; your workplace will have copies of these. If you are not aware of them, ask a senior person where they can be found. There may also be relevant legislation that could impact on the assessment process, including the Mental Health Act 2007, the Protection of Children Act 1999 and the Human Rights Act 1998. Your workplace will generally have a locally adapted version of these laws and it is your responsibility to make sure you have read the local policy and attended any training required.

Although we cannot explore these issues here in depth, you should familiarise yourself with the relevant laws. There are some further reading suggestions at the end of the chapter.

Ethical issues in assessment

As with all nursing care, assessment must be conducted ethically. Using the principles of biomedical ethics we must ensure:

- **beneficence** – take actions that promote the well-being of others;
- **non-maleficence** – do no harm;

- **justice** – work with a concept of moral rightness;
- **autonomy** – allow the patient to make informed and uncoerced decisions about his or her care as far as it is possible to do so.
  (adapted from Beauchamp and Childress, 2001)

Again, it is beyond the scope of this book to discuss ethics in detail, but you should be familiar with ethics from your other studies and apply them to the MH assessment (see the further reading at the end of the chapter).

Conclusion

Each person who needs to be assessed is unique; one of the things that makes mental health assessment so challenging *and* so interesting is its complexity. Although we have many assessment tools to guide and help us in our quest to assist our patients on their journeys to recovery, each situation will be slightly different and may require different skills from you. In this chapter we have outlined the principles of the process and important elements of an MH assessment. In the next chapter we will look at how we engage with the patient in order to help facilitate a good assessment.

Chapter summary

This first chapter begins to deal with several key issues; first is that it is important to know yourself well and be aware of the part you will play in shaping any assessment you are part of. Second, it is important to keep the patient at the centre of the assessment at all times and check that the care resulting from any assessment is in partnership with the patient and therefore the most likely to lead to a positive outcome for him or her on the pathway to recovery; we explore this in more detail in the next chapter. We have looked at some of the common principles of assessment and how they fit into the nursing process. We have also explored some of the practical, ethical, social, economic and legal issues of assessment along with issues of confidentiality. Assessment in mental health is a complex process made more so by the requirements of person-centred care, as there is no 'one size fits all' model and you must be guided both by patient need and your service expectations. Through a greater understanding of the nursing process, you will be able to develop a sense of how to nurse effectively and understand more clearly the knowledge, skills and values that a nurse contributes.

Activities: brief outline answers

Activity 1.2: Critical thinking (page 8)

In these definitions assessment is predominantly quantifiable and the suggestion is that we should be making judgements about the value or essential qualities of the person. This may sit uncomfortably with the expected stance of a mental health nurse as non-judgemental and person-centred.

The definitions by which we estimate the amount of any variable within an assessment situation, such as risk or levels of distress, should be judged by the standards of the patient not by the point of view of the nurse, thus highlighting the importance of keeping the patient's values at the centre of care.

Activity 1.5: Decision making (page 13)

You might say something like: 'Jim, before you do, as a healthcare professional, I must make it clear that there are certain things that I cannot keep confidential, such as risk to a child.'

If Jim indicates clear risks to himself or others, they must be shared.

Activity 1.6: Critical thinking (page 15)

Julie's values – A messy environment is an indicator that the inhabitant is low in mood; people should wash.

Some questions to ask – How often do you tidy your bedsit? How long have these beer cans been here? How much do you drink on a daily basis? Did you drink last night?

Greg may well feel completely undermined by the decision to keep him on the caseload and think that, in fact, he is still ill when he believed he was doing well and was on the path to recovery.

Further reading

Barker, PJ (2004) *Assessment in Psychiatric and Mental Health Nursing: In search of the whole person.* Cheltenham: Nelson Thornes.

This comprehensive book covers the theory of assessment and provides a solid foundation for practice.

Brown, R, Barber, P and Martin, D (2012) The Mental Capacity Act 2005, in *Mental Health Law in England and Wales*, 2nd edn (pp63–70). London: Sage.

This guide to the Mental Capacity Act provides some assistance in navigating the complicated legal framework.

Colliety, P and Horton, K (2012) Confidentiality, in Gallagher, A and Hodge, S (eds) *Ethics, Law and Professional Issues: A practice based approach for health professionals.* Basingstoke: Palgrave Macmillan.

This interactive chapter helps you to get to grips with the often difficult issue of confidentiality in practice.

Warner, L (2008) Identifying people's needs and strengths, in Stickley, T and Basset, T (2008) *Learning about Mental Health Practice.* Chichester: Wiley and Sons.

This chapter outlines the importance of working together in assessment and creating care packages and emphasises the requirement to identify individuals' strengths and capabilities.

Useful websites

www.dh.gov.uk/en/index.htm

This government website provides important information about current healthcare policy and data protection.

www.nice.org.uk

Search this website for guidance on all aspects of mental and physical healthcare.

www.time-to-change.org.uk

This website aims to end mental health discrimination and contains a wealth of useful resources including short films and blogs.

Chapter 2
Engaging the person

Yvonne Middlewick

NMC Essential Skills Clusters

This chapter will address the following ESCs:

Cluster: Care, compassion and communication

1. As partners in the care process, people can trust a newly registered graduate nurse to provide collaborative care based on the highest standards, knowledge and competence.

By second progression point:

6. Forms appropriate and constructive professional relationships with families and other carers.

2. People can trust the newly registered graduate nurse to engage in person centred care empowering people to make choices about how their needs are met when they are unable to meet them for themselves.

Chapter aims

By the end of this chapter you should be able to:

- define engagement in mental health nursing;
- understand the purpose of engaging with people using services and the relationship this has to the assessment process in mental health practice;
- reflect on your assumptions, values and beliefs and the impact these may have on building rapport;
- begin to understand the process of building relationships with people using mental health services.

Introduction

I recently asked three service users what they wanted most from the nurses working with them. They said that they wanted:

- to be listened to;
- to be treated with compassion;
- not to be spoken down to but to be treated as equals;
- people not to give up on them.

Building relationships with people is essential to being a mental health nurse, although it can be challenging when people are in distress. It is the foundation for developing a therapeutic relationship that can help people in their journeys through mental health services. The Nursing and Midwifery Council (NMC) emphasises the importance of these in the *Standards for Pre-registration Nursing Education* (NMC, 2010b) and *The Code* (NMC, 2008a).

This chapter explores how you build relationships with the people around you generally and within the context of mental health practice. You will also consider how nurses can build rapport with the people using their services, thereby enabling them to engage in the assessment process and begin their recovery journeys. We will bear in mind the four requests from service users, which are in line with what recent reports and policies are telling us (DH, 2011a; NICE, 2012; Schizophrenia Commission, 2012).

What is engagement in mental health nursing?

In mental health nursing, as with other fields of nursing, it is important that patients are involved in decisions relating to their care. If they are not involved or engaged in this process, the likelihood for success is significantly reduced. You may be able to ensure that, for example, they take their medication, attend support groups etc. while they are in an inpatient environment or indeed under a section of the Mental Health Act, but these do not last forever and therefore we need to consider what happens when there is no involvement of inpatient services. Once a patient is back in his or her own environment, perhaps with some community support, he or she needs to be able to manage personal needs either independently or with the support of a carer. This is a key time when patients can become disengaged from services, which may result in the re-emergence of mental health problems and either further inpatient experiences or the involvement of crisis resolution teams.

The overall aim of care should be to engage patients and their carers to enable them to self-manage their conditions, to be able to identify when their mental health is deteriorating and to take appropriate early action to prevent further deterioration. This recovery-focused approach empowers people to remain in control of their lives and manage their mental health issues (DH, 2011a; NICE, 2012; Schizophrenia Commission, 2012). The challenge for us as nurses is how to support our patients to reach the point where they may want to self-manage and this is another good reason why it is important to engage them in their care processes regardless of the services they are in contact with. This process can be achieved through good communication to promote collaboration with patients and their carers.

Activity 2.1   *Reflection*

Think about your personal life and the last time you successfully met someone for the first time. Take a few minutes to reflect on the situation and make a list of the following:

- the person's demographic, for example age, sex or ethnicity;
- the environment where you met;
- how you were both introduced or what made you start speaking to each other;
- what sort of things you talked about in the first five to ten minutes.

Keep your list for use in Activity 2.4.

An outline answer is provided at the end of the chapter.

Back to basics

A good starting point is to review the basics of communication. What is communication and how does it happen? Reece et al. (2006, p273) define communication as *one person who sends or transmits a message which is received by a second person*. Bach and Grant (2009) describe communication as a basic human need to enable the sharing of ideas. They recognise that, although we now have more varied and technical ways of communicating, the fundamental principles remain the same.

Communication can be both verbal and non-verbal, and can involve many of the special senses including hearing, vision and smell as well as other systems of the body. These include, for example, the nervous system, to interpret messages received via the eyes and ears etc., and the integumentary system if we are using touch as a method of conveying a message. Once you consider the complex nature of communication it can help you begin to understand how the receiver may interpret the messages that are sent differently, particularly if they are distressed. It is therefore important that the person transmitting the message checks the understanding of the receiving person as this can help to reduce misunderstandings. It can also help the person

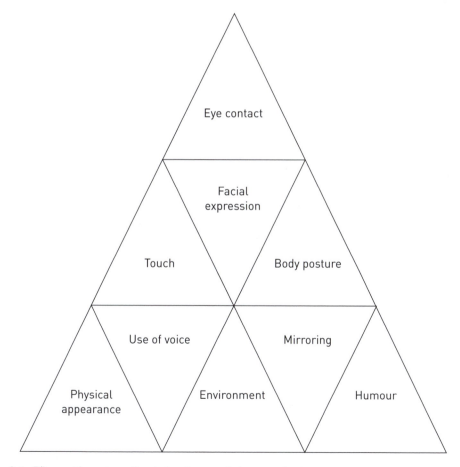

Figure 2.1: The complex nature of verbal and non-verbal communication.

Source: Adapted from Killick and Allan (2001, pp45–6).

assessing the patient to gain an understanding of his or her situation. For example, if a patient is hearing voices he or she may have difficulty concentrating and hearing the message you are trying to convey. It is important to consider how distressing this may be, particularly if the voices are abusive or critical. With this occurring it is perhaps understandable that the patient may find it difficult to listen to the person doing the assessment.

Activity 2.2   *Reflection*

Take a few minutes to think about your experience of working within the field of mental health. Make a list of the 'tools' you have used to help you care for your patients – for the purpose of this activity a 'tool' is interpreted as anything, formal or informal, that has helped you in assessing and planning care. These will be considered in Activity 2.4.

An outline answer is provided at the end of the chapter.

Basic but complex

Figure 2.1 outlines some of the basic requirements for good communication; however, this requires a complex interplay of both the people involved and the environment. This may be additionally more challenging when working with people with mental health problems as they may experience altered cognitive processes. This in turn may result in interpreting actions differently from when they are well. There are many books about communication skills but here are some areas of communication for you to consider within the context of mental health nursing.

Eye contact

Eye contact may seem like a simple aspect, but how do you ensure the right amount of eye contact? Too much and you may appear aggressive; too little and you may appear uninterested. You may find that some of your patients may use prolonged periods of eye contact and this can feel uncomfortable or aggressive when you do not know the person. Likewise, not looking at you may lead you to believe that they are not engaged with the interaction, which can feel equally challenging. You have to assess each person and decide what is comfortable for him or her every time you communicate. This is where experience helps you to interpret the behaviours of others and respond accordingly.

Mirroring

Once you are in tune with the other person you may naturally mirror his or her expressions and body language. This is deemed as good communication; however, it is important that you are self-aware as you do not want to mirror behaviours that may be considered aggressive as this may escalate a situation rather than make a person feel comfortable. Likewise, if you are assessing a person with depression you want to be empathetic but do not want to entirely 'mirror' his or her body language as you need to be able to engage the person and then draw him or her into the conversation. This will come with experience, as there will be times when your patient will not want to have a conversation with you. Remember that, in the introduction, service users said the important thing is to be treated with compassion and for people not to give up on them.

Physical appearance

Physical appearance is also an important element of communication. We make judgements about people from what they are wearing, their hair, jewellery and smell, for example. In policing, health work and other professions there are dress codes. These dress codes lead us to have a set of expectations about the behaviours of the profession. There is also the issue of recognition. In mental health nursing the issue of uniform generates much debate. From the 1970s many areas of mental health nursing felt that uniforms were a barrier to communicating with patients and decided that staff should wear their own clothes (Tham and Ford, 1995). However, in recent years many areas are starting to wear uniforms again. There does not appear to be any consensus about patients' views of uniforms, but what is clear is that they want to be able to identify staff and this can be done with a simple well-placed badge or identification card (Lefebvre, 2003; Sharkey, 2012; Tham and Ford, 1995).

Many patients in mental health nursing have altered cognition for a variety of reasons and this may affect their ability to recognise who is a nurse. An 80-year-old may also have very different expectations of what a nurse looks like. When such a person was younger, nurses probably wore dresses and hats, so a nurse in trousers and a polo shirt or tunic and trousers will not look like a nurse, particularly if the person has a condition affecting the memory. Additionally, because of their conditions, some patients may not recognise the nurse–patient boundaries.

Scenario

Imagine you are a registered community mental health nurse visiting a male patient, Jack, to give him a depot injection. You have visited him many times in the residential home where he lives. You go to his room and, as you are preparing the depot, he says that he just needs to get something. He rummages around on the shelf in his wardrobe and then he turns around with a thick fishing sock in his hand, which he holds out to you as he says 'here you are we will need this'. You are rather confused at this point. Jack looks exasperated and then says, 'do you want to put it on or shall I?' Totally confused now, you ask him why you need it and he states very matter of factly, 'you don't want to get pregnant do you?' At this moment you are stunned to realise that he has misinterpreted the reason for coming to his bedroom even though he appeared to understand at the time. You politely make your exit.

What would you do next?

The above scenario outlines how situations can catch you by surprise regardless of your experience and how well you may know the patient. Community mental health nurses tend not to wear uniforms and, although you may be dressed appropriately and in alignment with the local policy, misinterpretations can occur. It is important if this happens to discuss it with significant people so that you can gain support. In the case of the scenario this would be the residential home manager, your manager and your clinical supervisor.

Regardless of where you work there will be policies about how staff should dress. It is important that you follow them as these have been designed to help protect both you and your patient.

The use of touch

The use of touch is another valuable non-verbal skill. Touching can be a way of spontaneously connecting with a person and can be a comforting thing to do. Some people are happy to touch other people and to be touched themselves, but not everyone is comfortable with this. Nurses need to be mindful of how they are using touch and how it may be interpreted.

Activity 2.3   *Reflection*

- When you meet someone and they shake your hand, are you comfortable with a handshake?
- Do you prefer a firm handshake or a gentle one? If you prefer a firm handshake and then receive a gentle one in which the person hardly touches your hand, or the person has sweaty palms, how does that make you feel?
- Would you instigate a handshake with someone you meet for the first time? If not, why not?
- If you are comfortable with a handshake has this always been the case or has this developed? If so, how?

Consider your answers in light of the discussion below.

A handshake may seem a simple way to make contact by touch, but when you start to explore it you may find people have different preferences. We therefore need to be mindful that what is comfortable for us may not necessarily be the same for others. A handshake is a potential opportunity to reach out and make a physical connection with someone without it feeling too personal, but it could also feel very formal. If someone returns your handshake or chooses not to, it can give you an idea about how they are feeling at that time.

The use of voice

The use of our voices, which includes pitch, tone, intonation and pace of delivery, is a necessary consideration for both the assessor and the patient. Paying attention to these aspects of speech when listening to your patient may reveal that he or she is frightened, angry, upset, low in mood or euphoric. Patients may also make assumptions about you from the way you speak to them.

Keaschuk and Newton (2009) describe verbal communication skills that also demonstrate that you have listened as the ability to reflect, summarise or paraphrase. This also enables you to check with your patient that you have heard what he or she has said and to clarify that you have understood the meaning.

The mental health nursing context

Within mental health nursing communication is used to develop a relationship between the nurse and the patient. This is fundamental in enabling patients to become engaged with assessment and their care. Rask and Brunt (2007, p170) describe this relationship as *an interaction between nurses and patients based on contact and communication between two parties, where the patient is the focus*. They go on to describe the nurse as the tool to help the patient in distress through the development of a caring relationship (Rask and Brunt, 2007). Brown (2012, p21) suggests that in building a therapeutic relationship *we need to use who we are as a healing influence in our relationships with clients*. This is one of the unique qualities of being a mental health nurse compared with other fields of nursing. This is not to say that communication skills are not important to other nurses, or indeed all healthcare professionals, just that they often have additional tools in the form of equipment to help them successfully care for their patients.

Activity 2.4 *Reflection*

Compare your list from Activity 2.2 with the discussion above. How many items on your list involve a tool other than yourself? You may have put things such as risk assessment tools, nutritional assessment tools or one of the many rating scales that are available. However, these are heavily reliant on the communication skills of the assessor to encourage the patient to engage with the process to ensure that the assessment is accurately completed.

As this activity is based on your own list, there is no outline answer at the end of the chapter.

It could, however, be argued that, regardless of tools that are used to support patients in any field of practice, the nurse–patient relationship is not only fundamental in providing high-quality, person-centred care but a professional requirement (NMC, 2008a, 2010b). Peplau (1952) identified the importance of the nurse–patient relationship in the 1950s as being the foundation of supporting people and helping them to develop. Although this work may have been published a long time ago it is considered seminal and can be seen referenced in mental health literature. If you consider the foundations of providing a 'helping' rather than 'controlling' relationship, this can be linked to the type of relationships required to empower patients and enable a recovery-focused approach to care.

Barker (2009) suggests that there is a difference between the relationships needed to contain a crisis and those needed for longer-term growth and development. In the former it is the nurse's role to provide a safe and secure environment to protect the patient during a period of distress or to hold on to hope while the person is unable to hold on to this for themselves (Deegan, 1996). Once the period of crisis is over, this relationship should change to enabling collaboration and returning the 'hope' back to the patient. This relationship is likely to be longer and more sustained, but the foundations will be set early in the relationship. Consider the following case study.

Case study

John, a 35-year-old, has been admitted to a Psychiatric Intensive Care Unit (PICU). He has been brought to the unit in handcuffs escorted by four police officers following an incident in the town centre on a Friday night. He appears to be hearing voices and the police suspect that he has been drinking heavily and may have taken illicit drugs.

On arrival he is extremely aggressive to the staff and tries to leave the unit. His behaviour becomes threatening to staff. Following consultation with the team a decision is made that he should be restrained and given intramuscular medication in line with the rapid tranquillisation policy. The restraint team are organised and everyone is clear about their roles. Throughout, one member of the team speaks to John to keep him informed about what is happening and to assess his mood. As soon as he is calmer and the level of risk is reduced moves are made to gradually increase his level of independence.

Activity 2.5	Critical thinking

- Why do you think John was behaving aggressively?
- What impact could the restraint have on future relationships with John?

Consider your answers in light of the discussion below.

When John is admitted to the PICU in crisis there is a need to understand why he may be exhibiting this behaviour. It could be due to a number of reasons:

- hearing distressing voices;
- the effects of illicit drugs and/or alcohol;
- anger at the police for restraining him;
- anger at being brought to the PICU.

The reason for John's behaviour on this occasion was that he was frightened by a number of things: the voices he was hearing, the police, including the number of them bringing him in for admission, and the other patients in the PICU. Being frightened leads to stimulation of the neurobiological system, resulting in a complex series of events leading to a fight or flight response (Bear et al., 2007; Marieb and Hoehn, 2010).

In a PICU this can be difficult as the person may be unable to leave the situation and may not be able to articulate his or her fear, leading to the only other available option – to fight or behave aggressively. If the patient is then treated in a disrespectful and undignified way during a restraint, that can leave him or her with feelings of being frightened and aggressive towards the staff concerned. Even though John was in crisis on admission, being treated in a dignified, respectful and hopeful manner can help to begin to build a therapeutic nurse–patient relationship and lead to engagement in the care process.

Meeting patients for the first time (building relationships)

You may be meeting a patient or a group of patients for the first time because you are new to a clinical area or team. This can be a challenging time when you may feel you are a transient member of the team; however, it is important that you begin to build relationships quickly to enable you to gain confidence to contribute to the care of people in that area. You may be meeting someone for the first time in his or her home, which can feel very different as you are the visitor to that person's environment rather than him or her being a visitor to yours. Although you may be meeting the patient for the first time, it is likely that he or she may have met numerous professionals in his or her journey through mental health services.

Activity 2.6　　　　　　　　　　　　　　　　　　　　　　　　*Communication*

- Make a list of all the professionals you have encountered during your clinical practice experience. You may include those from healthcare, social care, the private and voluntary sectors and the criminal justice sector.
- Now think of a patient you have nursed and jot down all the professionals who were involved and their contribution to the care and treatment; you should include professionals who are not from mental health services, for example the GP, pharmacist etc. You might also consider whether any of the person's family were involved.

An outline answer is provided at the end of the chapter.

Once you start to think about how many people may have been involved in the care of one person you can begin to build up a picture of how many times that person may have told his or her story. Patients can become understandably irritated by having to say the same things to many different people. Having to do this also gives the impression that the lines of communication are not robust and this may not inspire confidence in patients or their families. There have been a number of high-profile cases in recent years that have highlighted poor communication across professions and organisations, leading to poor patient outcomes (Francis, 2013; Kennedy, 2000; Laming, 2003, 2009). The importance of communication in healthcare can never be overestimated in ensuring high-quality care.

NICE (2012) identifies that a professional completing a mental health assessment can act as either a facilitator or a barrier within the assessment process. It emphasises the importance of building trusting, respectful and empowering relationships in which patients feel valued and listened to. This requires nurses to provide both time and 'presence' to build this type of connection (Brown, 2012; NICE, 2012; Schizophrenia Commission, 2012). Heron (2001) enhances this further by suggesting that there is also a need for concern, empathy and genuineness.

Barker (2009, p8) suggests that it is the role of the nurse to be caring and that *caring emphasizes the caution, attention to detail and sensitivity necessary when handling something precious*. The author goes on to say that all people should be viewed as *priceless* (p8). If you treat everyone in this way and consider if your actions reflect how you would expect yourself or those close to you to be treated, this should help you when working with people with complex health needs. The skills outlined above do not necessarily require 'training' to achieve, but they are fundamental in building therapeutic relationships.

It can be difficult to build a trusting and empowering relationship if the patient feels as though you are asking hundreds of questions so that you can fill in your forms. Although assessment is clearly important, it is equally important to listen and be led in the conversation by the person. If you give a person the opportunity to tell his or her story, you can often find out the majority of information without having to ask all the questions. This can be achieved by asking open questions such as 'tell me about yourself' or, if you want to be more specific because of their distress, 'tell me about what has been happening to you that has led you to be here today'. Sometimes people don't want to talk about how they are feeling immediately, so getting to know them by finding out about the person more generally can help you to build a rapport. If you are also able to speak to a friend or carer it can help you build a picture of the person and his or her story. It is far easier to care for someone in a 'human' way if we can see the person behind the illness and distress. We are all complex beings and develop as a result of our experiences.

Activity 2.7   *Reflection*

Take a few minutes to consider the sort of information you would be willing to share with a professional you have just met.

- What would make you more likely to share personal information?
- What information would you definitely not share?

Consider your answers in light of the discussion below.

Some information is much easier to share, such as your name, age, job, if you are married or if you have children. You may also be willing to share things about your physical health, such as if you have your bowels open regularly (some people may not be feeling so keen at this point). However, if you have experienced physical, emotional or sexual trauma from an early age it may be very difficult to articulate this to someone you have just met, even if it is causing you a great deal of distress. It is therefore important to be led by the person, allowing him or her to talk about things that are comfortable for them.

Fredriksson and Lindström (2002) found that initially patients hide their suffering as a way of coping with it. Their research focused on the narratives of patients; however, they were able to identify that the skills needed by the nurse to enable the patient to share experiences was the ability to be present and listen sensitively. A number of authors stress the importance of the nurse demonstrating 'presence' in building therapeutic relationships (Brown, 2012; Fredriksson and Lindström, 2002; NICE, 2012; Schizophrenia Commission, 2012). This means that the nurse is actively involved in what the patient is saying rather than being distracted by other things that may need doing. During the time you spend with patients they should feel that they are the most important people to you.

Fredriksson and Lindström (2002) say that patients need to find their own 'turning point' to enable them to risk disclosing their distress to a third party. Patients having to reach a particular point when they are ready to disclose information is like the account of a recovery journey given by Deegan (1996). The important factor is that the patient needs to drive the change, which is supported by the practitioner. This is why you need to have conversations and a plan of care that is person centred. In summary, although we need to gather certain information so as to complete our assessment, we can gain this information in such a way as to develop our relationship with the patient. Let us now look at what can prevent the development of this relationship and thereby impact on the ability of the patient to engage with the assessment process.

Barriers to communication

Bach and Grant (2009) consider general barriers to communication in their chapter 'Understanding potential barriers'. The focus of their work is adult nurses; however, the generic barriers to communication are the same for mental health nurses. What mental health nurses also need to consider are the added complexities at communicating with clients who may be acutely distressed by their symptoms; for example, if someone is hearing voices, how can he or she be expected to focus on the conversation between you? Cognitive impairment, regardless of cause, can result in a distortion of the messages transmitted and received, leading to a situation in which communication becomes challenging.

Stories

Stories can be used to convey messages and information that are both fact and fiction and are often experienced and enjoyed throughout life. Within nursing, stories can be used to share experiences and the learning gained from these.

Case study

Sam was admitted to the acute unit in which Kate works as a registered nurse. Kate was trying to complete all the admission paperwork before the end of her shift as she did not want to hand it over to the night staff. Sam was not keen to answer any of the questions, which was proving frustrating for Kate. Having recently completed a course about person-centred care, Kate had been thinking about the telling of stories to help in getting to know patients. The suggestion was that nurses should have a blank piece of paper rather than assessment tools when building a relationship. Kate decided to put the paperwork away and to ask Sam to tell her about himself. Kate was surprised to find that this resulted in Sam telling her about his family and the fact he had written a book about his life in the armed forces. He also disclosed that his son was an

continued . . .

> *alcoholic who lived with him, and that his wife had committed suicide following the death of their daughter. Kate gained far more information about the context in which Sam lived. The things that were important to him were established during this conversation, which focused on the story he wanted to tell compared to the original task-orientated approach. This resulted in a relationship in which there was trust between Kate and Sam. Kate completed many of her assessments from the information Sam gave her during the telling of his story.*

While Fredriksson and Lindström (2002) describe how patients may conceal their distress when they first tell their stories, Lorem (2008) describes how staff can easily recall the details of stories they have been told by patients. He discussed the importance of using narratives for people who have psychosis as this can help us understand the patient's perspective. He goes on to state that narratives *may lead us to understand something valuable about very clear and real problems for the patient* (Lorem, 2008, p67). Therefore, allowing someone to tell his or her story can help us to understand why the person might be frightened, aggressive or withdrawn, enabling the nurse to gain insight from the patient's perspective.

Fredriksson and Lindström (2002, p403) state that the skilled dialogue that takes place between the nurse and the patient can enable *patients to, step by step, re-establish the interpersonal bridge*, providing a foundation for a good relationship to enable the sharing of experiences when the patient reaches his or her 'turning point'.

Conclusion

Communication takes various forms and is something that we do every day with the people around us. This may be happening in increasingly technical ways; however, it is important to ensure that we revisit basic communication skills to ensure that we understand the fundamentals of building a therapeutic relationship with patients who often have complex health needs. Skilled practitioners make building relationships look easy and this is because they spend years developing these skills. It is important to reflect on any challenging situations and accept feedback from colleagues, patients and their carers throughout your career. This will enable you to develop skills that are in alignment with your underpinning values, beliefs and professional requirements, so that you can truly be the nurse you want to be.

Chapter summary

In this chapter we looked at what engagement means in relation to mental health nursing. We then reviewed the basics of communication and went on to describe the complex nature of verbal and non-verbal communication, considering especially the cognitive processes involved and the fact that patients in mental health nursing may experience altered

continued . . .

cognition, thus making communication more challenging. Continuing on from this theme, we examined the development of the therapeutic relationship and its importance in the mental health nursing context, as well as the difficulties involved in the sharing of information. Finally, potential barriers to communication were considered, and the importance of narrative in the assessment of people in distress psychosis was stressed.

Activities: brief outline answers

Activity 2.1: Reflection (page 26)

There may be huge variation between your environment and the environment where you successfully met someone for the first time. The difference in age between you may also be quite significant. It is, however, likely that during the interaction you asked (or were asked) questions that enabled you to find some common ground. This may be an area of interest, for example football, gardening, cooking etc., or something related to your family, for example if you have children.

Activity 2.2: Reflection (page 28)

Some of the tools you may have chosen are: risk assessments, nutritional assessments, depression or anxiety screening tools, activities of living, the assessment of skin integrity, or screening tools for the use of substances. This list is not exhaustive and you may have identified many more.

Activity 2.6: Communication (page 33)

The areas you have been to on your clinical placements will influence the staff you have met. If you are at the beginning of your education, it is possible that you may not have an extensive list as perhaps your focus has been to understand your role as a nurse. As you progress there is an expectation that you will begin to recognise the contribution of other professions to the patient's journey.

From the patient's perspective have you considered the people involved at that moment in time or have you considered the longer-term involvement of people? For example, if you currently have a community experience perhaps you have only considered the involvement of the community mental health team, when perhaps your patient is also seeing his or her GP, carer, pharmacist, practice nurse, specialist nurses (e.g. if your patient has diabetes), podiatrist or psychiatrist. If there is also a physical health problem, the list begins to get even longer. Different people will also have been involved if the patient has come to your service through the criminal justice system.

Further reading

Barker, PJ (2009) *Psychiatric and Mental Health Nursing: The craft of caring* (2nd edn). London: Hodder Arnold.

This book provides practical advice from many areas of practice and is supported by service user perpectives.

Tee, S, Brown, J and Carpenter, D (2012) *Handbook of Mental Health Nursing*. London: Hodder Arnold.

This book will give you an overview of current aspects of mental health practice.

Useful website

www.mind.org.uk

This website offers an overview of service user perspectives as well as lots of other useful information relating to mental health.

Chapter 3
Types of assessment

Diane Carpenter

NMC Standards for Pre-registration Nursing Education

Domain 1: Professional values

4. All nurses must work in partnership with service users, carers, groups, communities and organisations. They must manage risk, and promote health and well-being while aiming to empower choices that promote self-care and safety.

9. All nurses must appreciate the value of evidence in practice, be able to understand and appraise research, apply relevant theory and research findings to their work, and identify areas for further investigation.

Domain 2: Communication and interpersonal skills

7. All nurses must maintain accurate, clear and complete records, including the use of electronic formats, using appropriate and plain language.

Domain 3: Nursing practice and decision making

1. All nurses must use up-to-date knowledge and evidence to assess, plan, deliver and evaluate care, communicate findings, influence change and promote health and best practice. They must make person-centred, evidence-based judgements and decisions, in partnership with others involved in the care process, to ensure high quality care. They must be able to recognise when the complexity of clinical decisions requires specialist knowledge and expertise, and consult or refer accordingly.

3. All nurses must carry out comprehensive, systematic nursing assessments that take account of relevant physical, social, cultural, psychological, spiritual, genetic and environmental factors, in partnership with service users and others through interaction, observation and measurement.

NMC Essential Skills Clusters

This chapter will address the following ESCs:

Cluster: Care, compassion and communication

6. People can trust the newly registered graduate nurse to engage therapeutically and actively listen to their needs and concerns, responding using skills that are helpful, providing information that is clear, accurate, meaningful and free from jargon.

Cluster: Organisational aspects of care

9. People can trust the newly registered graduate nurse to treat them as partners and work with them to make a holistic and systematic assessment of their needs; to develop a personalised plan that is based on mutual understanding and respect for their individual situation promoting health and well-being, minimising risk of harm and promoting their safety at all time.
11. People can trust the newly registered graduate nurse to safeguard children and adults from vulnerable situations and support and protect them from harm.

Chapter aims

By the end of this chapter you should be able to:

*   understand whether to read service users' notes before assessing them or not;
*   discuss the merits of comprehensive history taking and identify a history-taking structure;
*   evaluate universal, holistic, online and bespoke condition-specific approaches to assessment and evidence-based assessment tools;
*   critically debate the issues associated with involving service users meaningfully in their assessments.

Introduction

Paul arrived at the assessment unit overnight; his mental health nurse, Mohammad, meets him in the morning and is Paul's first contact with anyone from the mental health team. How Mohammad decides to assess Paul's needs is important for Paul's care and his well-being at the unit.

This chapter invites you to think more critically about assessment and to reflect on how it affects your practice. It will build on some of the reflective practice opportunities presented in Chapter 1. We will be discussing whether to read a patient's notes before undertaking an assessment, looking at history taking and learning to evaluate different kinds of assessment. In each of these areas, you can develop your critical thinking through reflecting on experience and considering the case studies presented.

Starting with the past or beginning with the present?

Some nurses will tell you that they never read a service user's notes before making an assessment; others will tell you that they always do.

Activity 3.1   *Critical thinking*

Think about the relative merits of reading a person's notes before or after making an assessment. Make a copy of the following table and complete it.

Benefits of assessment before reading a person's case notes	Benefits of reading a person's case notes before assessment
_____	_____
_____	_____
_____	_____
_____	_____
_____	_____
_____	_____
_____	_____

An outline answer is provided at the end of the chapter.

Once you have formulated your own ideas, take every opportunity to discuss the issue with other mental health practitioners from a variety of disciplines, especially those with differing lengths and types of experience. You may find that their thoughts are different from yours, and their ideas may help you formulate your opinion. If you are a novice practitioner, you may well benefit from listening to the experience of others and from broadening your perspective by talking to practitioners from other disciplines, even if you disagree with them.

There can be many reasons for not reading medical and nursing notes before assessing someone – including not wishing to be prejudiced by accounts of previous contacts with the service, or not wishing to form opinions based upon other practitioners' views of an individual. Just because someone has had several referrals or admissions for the same condition does not mean that the current presentation is the same. However, it would be foolish to miss important information, such as that which indicates the person we are about to assess could be at risk. There is no right answer to this, but in deciding you need to consider the context in which you will be making an assessment. If you are likely to be assessing someone you have not met before, or who may present a risk, then it would be wise to be aware of as much information as possible beforehand.

'Starting with the past', however, does not just mean reading a person's notes before assessment; it also means that we begin with the person's history rather than his or her current presentation. For people who are well known to the service, their long-term histories are probably fairly well documented, although this does not necessarily mean that they are comprehensive or current. You may wish to ask the person you are assessing to go over his or her history for clarification and expansion of details where possible. If, for instance, we decide not to ask someone about self-harming behaviour or previous suicide attempts, we might overlook important patterns that impact on the person's current presentation, even if that does not appear to be relevant to the person now. It also makes sense to ask the person you are assessing where he or she would like to begin. Sometimes people need or want to start with what has brought them here today. In any event you will need to be able to fill in the gaps in the person's written history to include his or her recent history, culminating in the assessment. History taking is an important skill and is integral to this chapter on types of assessment.

Most history taking follows a fairly standard format. Your place of work or clinical placement may use standardised case history forms either as paperwork or online questionnaires.

If you noted the history-taking format in your clinical placement it is likely that you will have identified the items listed below and suggested by Puri et al. (2002, pp68–70):

- reason for referral;
- present complaints (how is the person's problem affecting him or her?);
- history of presenting illness;
- family history;
- family psychiatric history;
- personal history: childhood, education, occupational history, psychosexual history, children, current social situation;
- past medical history;
- past psychiatric history;
- psychoactive substance use: alcohol, tobacco, illicit drug abuse;
- forensic history;
- premorbid personality (how would the person or his or her relatives describe the person's personality before he or she became unwell?).

Demographics will be addressed later in this chapter but form part of history taking. Barker (2004, pp70–2) suggests this is likely to include: age, sex and marital status, family, domestic situation, occupation, socialisation, financial status, personal belongings (where a person is being assessed for admission) and medication. Current presentation and factors relating to it are usually addressed fairly early on (history of presenting illness) and may include the following areas outlined by Barker (2004).

- **Functioning**: Are there any changes in physical functioning?
- **Behaviour**: Are there any recent changes in behaviour and are these affecting others or not?

- **Affect**: How does the person feel and are these feelings associated with the person's presenting problem?
- **Cognition**: What are the person's thoughts about his or her problems and how do these thoughts present themselves?
- **Beliefs**: What does the person believe will happen as a result of his or her problem(s)?
- **Physical**: Has the person experienced any associated physical problem?
- **Relationships**: Have his or her relationships with friends and family altered in any way recently (as a cause or consequence of the presenting problem)?
- **General orientation**: Is the person concerned about his or her view of reality?
- **Expectations**: What does the person think and/or hope will happen as a result of referral to the mental health services?

Now let us consider the following case study and ask whether we could address each of the topics included in taking a comprehensive history for Lucy, who we first encountered in Chapter 1 (see page 11).

Case study

Lucy is 20 years old and lives with her father. She is blonde, beautiful and has a great figure. Normally she is fairly introverted but generally friendly. She has a small group of supportive friends and a boyfriend of six months who is working at the local bank. She sees him about three times a week. They have recently become sexually active. She lost her virginity aged 18 to a previous boyfriend who wore her down to agreeing to sex even though she didn't feel ready. Her mother died of breast cancer when Lucy was 16. She gets on well with her father overall, although he drinks a lot more since the death of her mother and Lucy worries he may be addicted. She had some grief counselling at school when her mum died, but otherwise has no previous psychiatric history. She has no siblings. She does not feel she can confide in her dad as he is still obviously grieving for her mum and she does not want to add to his worries. She can talk to her boyfriend but they had a row recently because she was irritable due to being tired and she had criticised his driving skills. She is at university locally studying accounting and has been meeting her milestones academically. She does not know of any problems in her development and all her school targets were met.

Recently she has begun feeling very tired and wanting to sleep more than usual. She is very lethargic and describes dragging herself through each day like an automaton on a low battery. She feels very low and has not been eating – partly because she can't be bothered to cook. She has been finding it harder to concentrate and her reactions are slow. She was hit in the nose by a tennis ball recently when she was playing with a friend, which gave her a black eye. She stated that she felt her limbs were heavy and she couldn't reposition herself quickly enough to get out of the way. She has been complaining of low mood and lethargy so went to see the GP who has referred her to the practice mental health nurse for further assessment.

We know the *reason for her referral* by her GP was that Lucy had been complaining of low mood and lethargy and that her *present complaints* include her not feeling like cooking or eating and finding it hard to concentrate. The *history of her presenting illness* includes her having lost her virginity when not feeling ready, grief for her mother's death and concerns for her father and his alcohol intake, but other than this we have no further details about her *family history* or *family psychiatric history*. Lucy is at university and has a boyfriend so we can deduce something about her *education* and *social situation*, but other than that we know little of her *personal history*. We are not told anything about her *past medical history*, *past psychiatric history*, *psychoactive substance use* or whether she has a *forensic history*. We do, however, learn something of her *premorbid personality* in that she is normally fairly introverted, but generally friendly with a boyfriend and a small group of supportive friends.

We have a little information on her *physical functioning*, *affect*, *relationships* and *recent changes in behaviour*, but we are unaware of the rest of the factors associated with the history of her current presentation (*cognition*, *beliefs*, *physical problems*, *general orientation and expectations*).

This case study demonstrates the need to be thorough in taking a service user's history as part of the assessment process.

Online or bespoke?

Many kinds of assessment forms are available; some you can download from the internet either free of charge or at a cost. There are also those included in training packages for an individual or institutional fee, such as the *Camberwell Assessment of Need* (CAN) (Slade et al., 1999) (and its derivatives for specialist groups), which can be bought from the Royal College of Psychiatrists, who created it, and Steve Morgan's (2007) *Working With Risk Practitioner's* and/or *Trainer's Manuals*. Both of these are evidence-based – that is, they have been tested for validity and reliability so we can be reasonably confident in their likelihood of accuracy and of their being used and interpreted consistently by different practitioners. With such packages, purchase allows photocopying of the assessment tools and materials for training. With other assessment tools, for example the *Beck Depression Inventory* (BDI) (Beck et al., 1996), there are separate costs for the manual and assessment record/score sheets. These manuals and packages also tend to be evidenced-based. However, these do come at a cost, which is likely to be prohibitive to public organisations on a restricted budget.

This brief overview is likely to raise some questions, including the following.

- Are service providers' assessment processes evidence-based?
- Is it possible or allowable to mix assessment tools, e.g. to supplement an NHS Trust or service provider's assessment processes with a bespoke evidence-based tool (whether free or not)?
- Is there a perfect assessment tool with universal application or, if not, are there better assessment tools to assess certain mental health problems, needs or risks?
- What are the advantages and disadvantages of electronic assessment forms over paper ones?

Most Mental Health Trusts are now using electronic record systems, which incorporate the Trust's previous paper assessments and usually add in some specialist assessments as well, for example the *Historical-Clinical-Risk Management-20* (HCR-20) (Webster et al., 1997) for assessment of risk of aggression and violence. All NHS Mental Health Trusts have comprehensive risk policies that must be followed. These usually dictate the assessment formats considered acceptable and in most cases now these will be within an electronic system. So long as you complete the necessary assessments (whether they are in paper or electronic form) there is nothing stopping you supplementing your assessment by using more specific assessment tools if they appear to be useful. Examples may include the *Brief Psychiatric Rating Scale* (BPRS) (Overall and Gorham, 1962) or the *Edinburgh Postnatal Depression Scale* (EPDS) (Cox et al., 1987). These and other specific assessment instruments will be revisited later in this chapter.

One important aspect to consider, however, is the problem of overassessing service users. Some people may find being assessed intrusive, but necessary, whereas others may appreciate the time and care you spend in assessing them. Some assessments are written for the service user to self-assess, which may help supplement or be included in the formal process you have to take. In any event, throughout your career you are likely to come across new assessment tools; the important thing is to ascertain that they are valid and reliable, and to use them where appropriate – that is, where it may benefit the service user or provide you and the care team with a more comprehensive overview to help plan care and treatment. It is important, therefore, to consider whether the assessments used in the clinical areas in which you work are evidence-based. Many standard Trust-based clinical assessments have been developed over time, usually by senior staff from a variety of clinical backgrounds. These will not be evidence-based unless they have been tested through research processes. However, what is important in considering whether an assessment is evidence-based is the extent to which it is valid and reliable. Just because an assessment has not been through the formal research process to validate it does not mean that it is invalid or unreliable – just that we cannot know whether it is or not. But what is validity and reliability?

Validity and reliability in assessment tools

Bowling (2001, p21) maintains that validity is the extent to which the scale measures the underlying concept of interest. In other words, does it accurately measure what it sets out to measure? Tools need to have predictive validity; in other words, they should identify real changes in a condition, such as becoming more or less depressed, anxious or psychotic. They should also have social and clinical validity – that is, they should be sensitive to the social conditions relevant to the service user and identify fluctuations due to the condition and its treatment over time. Different aspects of validity should be measured in the process of determining the evidence base of an assessment instrument. These aspects of validity are:

- face validity;
- content validity;
- criterion validity;
- predictive validity;
- construct validity.

Activity 3.2   *Evidence-based practice and research*

Research the above five different aspects of validity and then select an evidence-based assessment tool – such as the Brief Psychiatric Rating Scale – and search for and read an article that discusses these aspects. Having done that, you will be able to approach other assessments with a critical eye before deciding whether you wish to use them in your clinical practice.

As this is an individual activity, there is no outline answer at the end of the chapter.

Holistic or specific?

Earlier in this chapter we asked whether there is a perfect universal assessment tool, but an assessment tool sufficiently comprehensive to be suitable to all people in all circumstances would be too long to complete both for the nurse and the person being assessed. An electronic assessment tool that would filter questions based upon the answers given would be useful, but is not currently available. The current electronic systems are a compromise.

It is important, however, to ensure that the assessment tool(s) you are using are suitable for the people you are assessing and you do need to amass comprehensive information in order to plan and provide holistic care. Currently a holistic approach is likely to be gained by assessing different specific areas and synthesising these in your formulation of care and care planning. For instance, in Lucy's case study, above, we might begin with the NHS Trust's standard holistic assessment tool, but because she shows signs of depression, we may use a specific assessment tool for depression such as the BDI II (Beck et al., 1996).

In Activity 1.1 (page 8) you were asked to consider what assessment meant to you and what would make you feel more or less comfortable in being assessed. You may like to review your findings, as the following activity develops this further.

Activity 3.3   *Communication*

You may like to undertake this exercise in pairs.

- Take a few minutes to consider what questions someone would have to ask you to find out the most about you.
- Write a list of them, and then asterisk the top five – those that would be the most useful to another person in getting to know the real you.
- Share your list with your friend or colleague and notice the similarities and differences.

Consider your answers in light of the discussion below.

This is an interesting question that has been tried and tested with hundreds of student nurses of all disciplines and the answers are always different. Some err perhaps on the side of caution when sharing their lists of questions and suggest only those that are least intimate or intrusive and say that name, age, occupation and address will reveal the most about them. Of course, these demographic variables are very important, particularly where someone lives, as this may provide some information about their socio-economic status and any environmental or neighbourhood risk factors. It is easy, however, to jump to conclusions about someone on the basis of our assumed knowledge. It would, though, lead to further questions. For instance, if someone told you they lived in a bedsit on a troubled housing estate, you would try to establish how the person came to be there, how long they had been there, whether their housing was adequate (dry, well-maintained with all the necessary amenities) with good neighbours or whether they were living in a damp, poorly maintained place with unfriendly or even abusive neighbours. It would not be hard to imagine that someone could well feel depressed, if not physically unwell, in such circumstances.

Other people answering this question come up with all sorts of questions that might reveal their true selves and some of the answers previously given include the following.

- Do you regularly read a newspaper and, if so, which one(s)?
- Which genre of literature/music do you most enjoy?
- How many friends/close friends do you have?
- Are you in a relationship and how would you describe it?
- Do you feel safe where you live?
- What is the most exciting/outrageous thing you have ever done?
- What do you regret most about your life?
- If you could change anything about your current circumstances what would it be?
- Have you ever been arrested?

You may question the wisdom of asking some of these questions very directly, but can probably appreciate how they (or versions of them) might begin to help engage with a person and get to know him or her better. Knowing a person better helps us to choose more specific questions that could be helpful. This is where generic demographic questions can lead to more person-centred questions; these in turn can lead to identifying further areas for specific assessment. For example, if you ascertained that someone was living in very poor housing you may well consider a needs assessment most pertinent.

We now return to one of the people you met in a Chapter 1 case study (see page 15). Greg is 34, lives alone in a bedsit and is being supported by the crisis team through a particularly difficult bereavement. He is visited by a nurse working in the crisis team who is to assess him for discharge. He is unwashed, his bedsit is a mess and there are many empty beer cans lying around.

Thinking about Greg's social situation you might list everything you feel it would be useful to know about him to be able to work with him most successfully and appropriately.

You may well consider the following questions.

- How long has he lived in the bedsit?
- In what sort of area is the bedsit situated?

- Is the bedsit unkempt because of Greg's mental state or is he battling with a poorly maintained environment?
- Are there any safety issues with the locality?
- Does he have any neighbours he talks to?
- Is he ever visited by friends or relatives?
- What is his financial situation?
- Does Greg work/is he off sick?
- If he is unemployed – how long has this been for? Is his unemployment because of his depression or made worse by it?
- How much alcohol does Greg drink?
- Has Greg started drinking because of his bereavement or did he drink before?
- To what extent is Greg's drinking exacerbating his depression?
- Did Greg's drinking contribute to his losing his job or did he begin drinking because he became unemployed?
- Has Greg got a washing machine or would he have to travel to a launderette to do his washing?
- Has Greg neglected his nutrition?
- How is Greg's physical health?

Having started with demographic details about Greg it is likely that you will have quickly progressed to identifying details that will contribute to his overall assessment and that will flag up more specific assessments, for example the CAN (Slade et al., 1999).

Greg's case may have raised several issues for you – not least concerns about his physical health. The Government's strategy for mental health, *No Health Without Mental Health* (DH, 2011a), outlines six key objectives, the third of which is: *that more people with mental health problems will have good physical health and that fewer people with mental health problems will die prematurely.*

Physical health assessment for people with mental health problems

Often the physical health needs of, problems of and risks to people with mental health conditions are overlooked and this group of people is more likely to die prematurely from a physical condition that could potentially have been identified and treated sooner. This is called *diagnostic overshadowing* and occurs in all areas of healthcare – not just mental health. For instance, minor health problems in pregnant women are frequently ascribed to the pregnancy and not fully investigated. Those with mental health problems may experience symptoms of an underlying health problem that mirrors side effects of their medication. For example, taking diazepam for anxiety might cause gastro-intestinal disturbances, but these might also indicate a gastric problem, such as an ulcer, which is not uncommon among those experiencing chronic anxiety or stress.

There is a myriad of health-related assessment tools and questionnaires. Electronic or paper assessment tools in clinical areas will include health-related questions, but it makes sense to be aware of further, more specific tools that might be used should a person complain of physical ill health. Below is a short list of some common assessment tools for health-related conditions:

- **General Health Questionnaire (GHQ)** (Goldberg and Williams, 1988);
- **Malnutrition Universal Screening Tool (MUST)** (Malnutrition Advisory Group, 2008);
- **Waterlow pressure ulcer scoring system** (Waterlow, 2008);
- **Diabetes Impact Measurement Scales (DIMS)** (Hammond and Aoki, 1992).

Activity 3.4   *Evidence-based practice and research*

- Read about the physical assessment scales listed above and establish what is known about their validity and reliability.
- Look up assessment scales for other health-related problems you have come across with people you have cared for.

As this is an individual activity, there is no outline answer at the end of the chapter.

In mental health nursing we do not generally assess physical health-related issues for the purposes of diagnosis, although we should identify symptoms of concern to discuss with our medical colleagues. Rather, we work with individuals in our care to assess the extent of the severity of symptoms and their impact on a person's life. Most of the assessment tools you will have discovered are focused on the quality of life issues for people suffering certain physical conditions.

Physical disease, however, is not the entire focus of physical assessment for people with mental health problems. Additionally, we aim to discover whether people are leading healthy lives, which may:

- identify risk factors for physical conditions and thus prevent disease processes from occurring;
- aid recognition of the severity of symptoms of existing conditions and therefore help to alleviate them;
- help to manage the side effects of some medications (e.g. weight gain).

Physical symptoms, conditions or states associated with mental health problems are also of particular concern. The areas in Table 3.1 are ones to note particularly.

Returning to Greg's situation, let us consider which aspects of his physical health we might wish to assess.

- *Sleep* – If he is depressed his sleep is likely to be disrupted. His alcohol consumption may also impact on this and possibly confound it.
- *Appetite* – Depression usually reduces appetite, which could lead to malnutrition. If his alcohol use is significant, he might be vitamin B1 deficient and require supplements.
- *Energy and activity* – We have no information about this, but a low mood is likely to mean that Greg is lacking energy and motivation. He may not be having fresh air and exercise, which is likely to make him feel more depressed. Additionally, lack of exercise and a poor diet, as well as psychomotor retardation from depression, could lead to constipation, which is likely to make him feel more sluggish and could also cause him to be confused.

Physical symptom	Specific relevance to those with mental health problems
Sleep	Difficulty getting off to sleep or early morning waking may be associated with depression and/or anxiety.
Appetite and nutrition	May be reduced in depression and anorexia nervosa, but increased in other eating disorders.
Energy and activity	May be reduced in depression and as a result of some medications and misuse of some substances, or increased in elated states and with other substance misuse.
Restlessness	Agitation and restlessness in depressed individuals is associated with an increased suicide risk; restlessness from an elated mental state puts the sufferer at risk of cardiac problems.
Pain	Chronic pain is associated with increased suicide risk.
Skin integrity	Older adults in particular may have very delicate skin at risk of pressure sores or ulcers.
Weight/obesity	Often results from anti-psychotic medication – puts the person at increased risk of all obesity-related health problems such as heart conditions and some cancers.
Hygiene	Poor hygiene is often a symptom of depression, psychotic conditions or dementia and puts people at risk of developing infections as well as making them more likely to be stigmatised.

Table 3.1: Important physical symptoms associated with mental health problems

- *Restlessness* – It seems unlikely that Greg is restless, but if he were found to be, that would be a risk factor for suicide.
- *Pain* – Is there any evidence that Greg has pain? If he is drinking to excess and eating a poor diet he may have gastro-intestinal problems causing him pain.
- *Skin integrity* – We know that Greg is unwashed – his skin could be affected by this and poor nutrition.
- *Weight/obesity* – Although there were empty beer cans lying around in Greg's flat, there was no account of any food remains – whether home cooked or take-away. He is more likely, therefore, to be underweight rather than overweight (although not necessarily so) and an assessment might need to be made of his nutrition and his weight might need monitoring.
- *Hygiene* – See *skin integrity* above.

It is likely that further assessment and management and/or care of Greg's mental state would impact significantly on his physical health. If he were not depressed he would possibly be less likely to drink alcohol and more likely to care for his physical health needs, which in turn would improve his mood further. Thus, while assessment needs to be truly holistic, specific and specialist assessments can contribute to this. While it is unlikely that there will be a comprehensive assessment tool to identify all of the factors relevant to Greg, using specific tools can help so long as the results from each are synthesised into a meaningful whole – that is, they are summarised and inform care planning.

Practitioner or service user perspectives?

Assessments may be designed to be completed by the clinician, by the service user, in consultation with a carer or any combination. It is usually good practice, where possible, to engage a service user fully in the assessment. A criticism of this approach is that clinicians may display tokenism rather than true collaboration with service users, so it is worth considering this critically. In other words, either engage the service user in a genuine way or not at all.

Activity 3.5   *Critical thinking*

Make a copy of the table below and use it to identify reasons for and against actively involving service users and carers in the assessment process. You may also wish to add in arguments you have heard from other practitioners. When you have done this, look carefully at your lists and consider whether your ideas could be challenged and possibly changed.

Reasons to actively involve service users/carers in the assessment process	**Reasons to exercise caution in engaging service users/carers in assessments**	**Can you challenge these thoughts?**
_____	_____	_____
_____	_____	_____
_____	_____	_____
_____	_____	_____
_____	_____	_____
_____	_____	_____
_____	_____	_____

Consider your answers in light of the discussion below.

It is likely that you identified many reasons for actively engaging service users and carers in the assessment process; however, you may have thought of some compelling reasons not to, or may have some concerns about doing so. It is those we will look at next.

Barriers to service user engagement

A service user may be intoxicated (in which case it is unlikely that anyone will be able to complete much of an assessment thoroughly). Also, a person may be acutely psychotic. Again, you and the service user would be challenged to complete all aspects of the assessment, although you may well be able to complete a mental state assessment based on your observations and the person's responses. It is important, however, not to assume that, because someone is very deluded or hallucinated, he or she cannot contribute to the assessment process. The person's expression of his or her experiences and beliefs should be taken seriously and noted. Service users may also be reluctant to disclose information for a variety of reasons – they might not know you and you may not yet have formed a therapeutic relationship; or they might be embarrassed, particularly if in the presence of loved ones/carers. In this instance you might offer to see them separately. You could consider giving service users a self-assessment form where this might be helpful – for example, the BDI (Beck et al., 1996).

Some service users might be suffering from cognitive problems, including failing memory. In this situation it is important to be as inclusive as possible, but you will need to verify a person's answers with someone who knows him or her well. Finally, you may not be sure whether someone is being totally honest with you. It is not uncommon for any of us to be economical with the truth on occasions, particularly if asked questions about our lifestyles, which we may not wholly want to own up to. Sometimes you will want confirmation from another person where serious issues are in doubt. On other occasions you may well be able to work with the service user's account and hope that, when you have developed a therapeutic relationship, he or she will come to trust you sufficiently to disclose more openly and reliably to you.

This is not an exhaustive list but indicates that there may be occasions where you might well be in doubt about a person's contribution to his or her own assessment, although our default position should always be to include rather than exclude. Assessments usually focus on problems, needs or risks and we can consider these with respect to service user/carer involvement. Carers or loved ones and clinicians may have completely different ideas from those of the service user about identifying problems, needs or risks. Although someone may be behaving bizarrely because of paranoid or grandiose delusions, he or she may not experience this as a problem. The person's loved ones, neighbours or society in general may have more of a problem with unusual, erratic or antisocial behaviour. If we as clinicians identify that a person has particular needs, but the person disagrees, he or she will be less likely to engage with any therapy or treatment offered. Conversely, if a person feels he or she has a particular need, but the care team disagrees, the person is likely to be left feeling frustrated and disappointed with the service. When considering risk assessment of someone who has recently tried to commit suicide, and the person tells you that he or she is glad to have survived and no longer feels like dying, the person may be not be telling the truth. It is quite possible for someone to say what he or she thinks the person completing the risk assessment wants to hear – in order to be discharged so that he or she can make another suicide attempt.

Assessment, whether of problems, needs or risks, is challenging and requires excellent engagement skills, empathy and the ability to focus on what people say and observation of how they say it – their non-verbal behaviour. The range of assessment tools is too numerous to itemise them all, but the next section identifies some that you are likely to find particularly useful.

Assessment toolkit

The following assessment tools are of particular note:

- **Beck Depression Inventory II (BDI-II)** (Beck et al., 1996);
- **Brief Psychiatric Rating Scale (BPRS)** (Lukoff et al., 1986);
- **Edinburgh Postnatal Depression Scale (EPDS)** (Cox et al., 1987);
- **Generalised Anxiety Disorder Assessment (GAD-7)** (Spitzer et al., 2006);
- **General Health Questionnaire (GHQ)** (Goldberg and Williams, 1988);
- **Geriatric Depression Scale (Short Form) (GDS)** (Hoyle et al., 1999);
- **Hamilton Anxiety Scale (HAS)** (Hamilton, 1969);
- **Instrumental and Expressive Functions of Social Support (IEFSS)** (Ensel and Woelfel, 1986);
- **Patient Health Questionnaire (PHQ-9)** (Kroenke and Spitzer, 2002);
- **Positive and Negative Syndrome Scale (PANSS)** (Kay et al., 1988).

You will notice that many of the assessment tools in the list above are quite dated now. This does not necessarily mean that they have no currency, however. Several of the assessments are for similar conditions, for example the HAS and the GAD-7 are both used to assess anxiety. It is worth considering the extent to which social change may have affected the currency of the HAS when compared with the more contemporary GAD-7. We should also consider the context in which it is to be used. In the 1960s and 1970s more people with mental health problems were cared for in hospital compared with today's trend for community-based services. It is important that we are satisfied that the assessment tools we use to aid our practice are serviceable in changing service environments.

Chapter summary

This chapter has offered the opportunity to consider critically whether or not to read service users' notes before assessing them. It has considered the merits of comprehensive history taking and identifying a history-taking structure, and has discussed the relative merits of universal/holistic online and bespoke condition-specific assessments. It has facilitated critical debate about the issues associated with involving service users meaningfully in their assessments and has signposted the reader to evaluate a range of evidence-based assessment tools in relation to contemporary clinical practice. In drawing the reader's attention to a range of assessment tools, it is important to remember that the therapeutic relationship and engagement with service users and carers is paramount and that the practitioner is more than the sum of his or her toolkit.

Activities: brief outline answers

Activity 3.1: Critical thinking (page 41)

Benefits of assessment before reading a person's case notes

- Avoids bias from previous reports.
- Avoids diagnostic overshadowing (the service user is assessed anew rather than in relation to his or her diagnosis).
- Promotes a more equal relationship with both parties meeting for the first time (where they have not met before).
- Allows the nurse's first impressions to be included as part of the assessment, which may give insight into how the person presents to others. Written information may distort these impressions.

Benefits of reading a person's case notes before assessment

- Avoids repetition of known details about the person, e.g. demographic information such as age and medical and psychiatric history.
- It may save time, which could be beneficial to the service user if he or she is particularly distressed or unwell.
- It may indicate any areas of known risk, which may help to protect the service user, the assessor or fellow service users.
- Previous care plans may indicate what the person being assessed finds useful and supportive.

Further reading

You may wish to read articles about the evidence base of assessment tools. The following two books may be of considerable help in this. Both books critique tools for assessing either particular 'diseases' or conditions or health status.

Barker, PJ (2004) *Assessment in Psychiatric and Mental Health Nursing: In search of the whole person*. Cheltenham: Nelson Thornes.

Note in particular appendices A and B in Barker's book. Appendix A addresses the research development of assessment instruments and Appendix B provides a selective bibliography of psychosocial assessment.

Bowling, A (2005) *Measuring Health* (3rd edn). Maidenhead: Open University Press.

Read this in addition to Bowling (2001) from your reference list.

Greenhalgh, T (2010) *How to Read a Paper: The basics of evidence-based medicine* (4th edn). Chichester: Wiley-Blackwell.

This book is really useful for critiquing research papers and can therefore be used to critique research related to assessment. In particular see Chapter 8, which provides a checklist for a paper that claims to validate a diagnostic or screening test. This could be applied to research papers that support the development of assessment tools.

Morgan, S (2007) *Working with Risk Practitioner's Manual*. Brighton: Pavilion Publishing.

This workbook provides a framework for assessing and managing risk and places the engagement of the service user's views and experiences as the foundation for collaborative risk working.

Useful websites

www.bapen.org.uk

This website raises awareness and understanding of malnutrition and its assessment. It gives further detail of the MUST tool.

www.patient.co.uk/doctor/Patient-Health-Questionnaire-(PHQ-9).htm

and

www.patient.co.uk/doctor/Generalised-Anxiety-Disorder-Assessment-(GAD-7).htm

These two links from the Patient.co.uk site provide a brief overview of the PHQ- 9 and GAD- 7 assessment tools mentioned in this chapter. They include copies of the assessment tools, which are free to use, and suggest further reading. The articles are written for healthcare professionals.

Chapter 4
Challenges to assessment

Sandra Walker

NMC Essential Skills Clusters

This chapter will address the following ESCs:

Cluster: Care, compassion and communication

5.   People can trust the newly registered graduate nurse to engage with them in a warm, sensitive and compassionate way.

By entry to the register:

10.   Has insight into own values and how these may impact on interactions with others.

11.   Recognises circumstances that trigger personal negative responses and takes action.

6.   People can trust the newly registered graduate nurse to engage therapeutically and actively listen to their needs and concerns, responding using skills that are helpful, providing information that is clear, accurate, meaningful and free from jargon.

Cluster: Organisational aspects of care

9.   People can trust the newly registered graduate nurse to treat them as partners and work with them to make a holistic and systematic assessment of their needs; to develop a personalised plan that is based on mutual understanding and respect for their individual situation promoting health and well-being, minimising risk of harm and promoting their safety at all times.

Chapter aims

By the end of this chapter you should be able to:

*   describe many of the challenges that can affect assessment in mental health nursing;
*   demonstrate a deeper understanding of the effect of social influences on the assessment process;
*   list basic ethical issues that apply to the assessment process;
*   take actions that can begin to address challenges of assessment in mental health practice;
*   begin to understand some of the ways common risks can impact on the assessment.

Introduction

Scenario

Late one evening you are called to assess Jade, a 15-year-old girl who has expressed suicidal ideas. She is there with her mother, who insists on being present. Jade keeps her back firmly towards her mother throughout the assessment and answers all your questions with either yes, no or a swear word.

Even a straightforward assessment in mental health nursing can be complex and there are many challenges that can make the process even more difficult. These range from practical problems, such as having no private room to conduct an assessment in; to ethical issues, such as having to break confidentiality in risk situations; to communication problems, such as Jade's; to social problems, such as patients stating there are no problems with their mental health as they are worried about the social stigmatisation it would cause if they were to be supported by mental health services.

The purpose of this chapter is to consider some of the problems you may encounter in carrying out assessments in mental health nursing and help you to see some potential solutions that may help you in overcoming the challenges you may confront when in practice. Of course, each patient is unique, with different problems, social background and needs, so the challenges that arise for each assessment will be different. So this chapter cannot cover every eventuality but many of the most common problems are addressed.

This chapter will first revisit some of the political, technical and legal issues we encountered in Chapter 1, then look in more detail at the economic issues that can challenge our assessment. The social and cultural impact of assessment is considered next, with a closer look at how stigmatisation can affect self-perception and the intricacies of involving family and carers in the assessment process. The chapter then moves on to consider some of the ethical issues that can become a challenge in the assessment process, with a further look at practical challenges, including talking to people who are highly emotional. We finish this chapter by considering some of the risk issues that may pose a challenge to assessment.

Political, technical and legal challenges to assessment

We began to consider these aspects in Chapter 1 and here we look at some of them in a little more detail.

NICE guidance

Much of the condition-specific guidance provided by NICE contains information designed to help in assessment of people with mental health; however, it is not always easy to spot.

Activity 4.1 *Critical thinking*

Read the quick reference guidance from the NICE website (www.nice.org.uk) on anxiety and borderline personality disorder (BPD).

- What information is given here to assist with assessment?
- Is it clear?

Outline answers are provided at the end of the chapter.

It is often necessary to interpret these documents in light of the task you have to do, as they are very general in nature and are designed to give a baseline standard that everyone offering care in these areas should conform to.

NMC guidelines

We discussed the NMC guidelines for confidentiality in Chapter 1. However, there are other points within the NMC *Code* (2008a) that affect us in our role as mental health nurses carrying out assessments.

Activity 4.2   *Critical thinking*

Find and read a copy of the NMC document, *The Code: Standards of conduct, performance and ethics for nurses and midwives* (www.nmc-uk.org/Publications/Standards).

- What information does it give that would impact on your role when carrying out a mental health assessment?

An outline answer is provided at the end of the chapter.

We have already discovered the importance of treating people as individuals, respecting confidentiality, collaborating with patients, working with other professionals in order to provide high-quality care, being honest and open, and keeping accurate records of the assessment. In carrying out a good assessment you will be adhering to the code of practice, which makes it more likely that you will be providing high-quality care even when you are unable to meet the needs of the patient concerned due to lack of resources.

Economic challenges to assessment

At the time of writing we are facing one of the most challenging times in healthcare in terms of financial constraints. The white paper, *Equity and Excellence: Liberating the NHS* (DH, 2010a), and the *Operating Framework* (DH, 2011b) both stress the importance of managing the decreasing financial resources available to the NHS in such a way that we must be more productive for less money. While this poses many ethical dilemmas in itself, which we cannot discuss here, the reality is that it can mean there are not the resources to which we can refer people when they need further treatment or support. In this instance it becomes important to be aware of self-help material that the person can access themselves, hopefully facilitating their own recovery without using NHS resources. Additionally, a working knowledge of the voluntary and non-statutory agencies, for example the Samaritans, is essential as these organisations are often the ones most likely to provide follow-up care for patients with mild to moderate needs. The National Institute for Health and Care (formerly Clinical) Excellence (NICE) is tasked with making decisions about treatments that have high cost and sometimes states that certain patient groups are not allowed to receive treatment for some conditions.

> ## Activity 4.3   *Evidence-based practice and research*
>
> - Go to the NICE website (www.nice.org.uk) and find the guidance on dementia care. Read this and see where the guidance makes specific statements about which treatments should be allowed and at what stage of the illness.
> - Following this, do a web search regarding the press coverage of the guidance when it was released.
>
> *As this is an individual activity, there is no outline answer at the end of the chapter.*

The assessment is an essential part of healthcare in that it helps us to decide, with the patient, the correct course of his or her recovery journey. Getting this right is important both from the point of view of patient need and also so as not to waste resources. If we get the assessment right first time it will inevitably be more efficient and effective. Therefore, it is very important to listen to patients' viewpoints and allow them to have an active role in the decisions made wherever possible. In Chapter 1 we considered false negatives and false positives in assessment and the results in terms of unnecessary patient treatment and ensuing costs. Overassessment and duplication of assessment are also considerations in our battle to be efficient and effective. Do not overburden patients with questions that they have already answered.

Social challenges to assessment

Research summary: Assessing the mental health needs of older adults from diverse ethnic backgrounds (Rose and Cheung, 2012)

This study was conducted to provide additional evidence to inform those constructing the new *Diagnostic and Statistical Manual* (DSM-5) and ensure that the challenges inherent in the assessment of older people of black and minority ethnic (BAME) cultures were considered appropriately. The study highlighted some of the major challenges found in assessing this patient group, including the following:

- a reluctance of BAME older people to admit to mental health issues due to embarrassment or shame;
- BAME older people denying or misrepresenting problems even once they are receiving care;
- cultural beliefs about services being inadequate and more effective for their white counterparts;
- clinicians often not being culturally competent and not understanding the cultural expectations and pressures that affect BAME older people;
- language barriers impacting on effective communication.

Method

A literature search was conducted looking at the processes and limitations of assessment for BAME older people; 54 articles were identified that had been published between 2001 and 2011. This included 28 research-based articles and 26 editorials, commentaries and literature reviews. Keywords were drawn from this selected literature and thematically discussed, and issues of quality were considered for each article.

Findings

Five main themes emerged.

1. **Assessment issues related to acculturation**
   When a person moves from one culture to another he or she may have trouble adapting. Of concern is the possibility that treatment may be applied without considering the person's traditional cultural values. If the assessor is not culturally competent it is likely that this could increase distress for the patient. For example, asking a family member to interpret may restrict the answers a patient gives in an assessment situation as he or she does not wish to be embarrassed in front of a family member by admitting to mental health problems.

2. **Limitations with cultural elements**
   There are some disorders that are uniquely cultural, for example *taijin kyofusho* – a social phobia common in Japan, and these are not considered in the literature. BAME older people are much more likely to attend the doctor with a somatoform disorder due to cultural tendencies to suppress mood and negative feelings. If a depression is believed to have occurred for biological reasons, for example hypothyroidism, the older person is more likely to seek help than if he or she blames the mood change on social or personal factors such as social isolation.

3. **Health disparities**
   BAME older people do not always have the knowledge to enable recognition of a mental health problem should one develop. This is of particular concern as mental health issues are often more severe in older adults. There is also the possibility that those who have come from a culture of stigmatisation and traumatic events may be reluctant to trust professionals, thus making it difficult to assess them and identify any treatment that may be required.

4. **Evidence-based practice in specific diagnoses**
   There is an identified lack of professional knowledge regarding evidence-based practice that should underpin the practice of professionals in this area; of particular concern is the lack of knowledge relating to dementia.

5. **Prevalence of anxiety and depression**
   Depression is often underreported in BAME older people and the services available are based on the needs of white older people and, therefore, may not be appropriate for

BAME older people and this may discourage them coming forward to access support. Many cultures traditionally rely on the wider family for support where mental health issues arise, but with an increase in migration this support is eroded, compounded by newer generations of the same family growing up in the new culture and not necessarily adopting the traditions of the originating culture.

Recommendations for practice

It is essential to ensure that staff are culturally competent, so training is required to close the gaps in their knowledge. It is also essential to be aware that BAME older people may have even higher levels of guilt and shame associated with suffering from mental health issues than the general population and this may affect reporting. More research is needed to ascertain the cultural differences in the expression of mental illness and culturally specific diagnoses. The study concluded that additional consideration of ethnic, cultural and gerontological issues needed to be incorporated into subsequent updates of the DSM.

From this research summary we see that several social challenges come into play. The notion of stigmatisation related to mental health can have a serious impact on the uptake of mental health services. This can range from the fear of family prejudice or shame to the change of personal identity that can result from having a mental illness. The difficulty of involving family and carers in the treatment of a person with mental illness is fraught with difficulties and can have a serious impact on the person's recovery.

Ethical challenges to assessment

The role of the mental health nurse is often underrated. The importance of giving high-quality care is as important as giving the correct treatment. It is well documented that patients report higher satisfaction levels if the care received from staff is compassionate and respectful. As this is the case and in alignment with the NMC *Code* (2008a), mental health nurses must strive to be ethical at all times. Every relationship with a patient, however fleeting, has the potential for healing and this creates a responsibility for nurses in their conduct both professionally and personally.

There are many ethical theories that impact to varying degrees on healthcare practitioners and this book cannot cover them all, and you will no doubt be drawn to some more than others depending on your own core values.

Duty-based theory – deontology

Deontology is primarily concerned with the duties or obligations inherent on a person doing what is morally right. The philosopher most closely connected to this theory is Immanuel Kant (1785). This theory is a key one when it comes to influencing professional codes of conduct.

Consequence-based theory – utilitarianism

Utilitarianism is an ethical theory which holds that the correct course of action is the one that maximises the overall 'good' of the greatest number of people. It is therefore a form of *consequentialism*, which means that the moral worth of an action is determined by its outcome. The most influential contributors to this theory are considered to be Jeremy Bentham and John Stuart Mill (Mill, 1861).

Virtue-based theory – biomedical approach

This theoretical approach is the one that has the most impact on healthcare and we have already met the first four of these principles in Chapter 1. The most important values that commonly apply to medical ethics discussions are:

*   **autonomy** – the patient has the right to refuse or choose their treatment;
*   **beneficence** – a practitioner should always act in the best interest of the patient;
*   **non-maleficence** – first, do no harm;
*   **justice** – concerns the distribution of increasingly scarce health resources, and concerns fairness and equality;
*   **dignity** – the patient (and the person providing treatment) have the right to be treated with dignity;
*   **truthfulness and honesty** – the concept of informed consent has increased in importance since the Second World War.

Rights-based theory

This theory is relatively modern and is based around the assumption that people have individual rights according to national or international rights frameworks. It is very culturally variable since there is no point in asserting that everyone has a right to demand good healthcare as some cultures still do not offer a healthcare service.

Case study

Gwen is 64 years old and has a history of depression. She has been a patient of community mental health services for over a year and is very isolated. She has one son, Graham, who has control of her finances and visits her regularly. There is some evidence that her son is cheating her out of her pension and he has become violent towards her in the past. It is believed that, as a vulnerable adult, she is at risk from her son and you have been asked to assess the extent of the problem. Upon discussion Gwen discloses that she is aware that he is cheating her out of money but prefers not to address it as she fears being left completely alone. You are acutely aware that her son is behaving illegally.

- As the nurse involved with Gwen, decide on a course of action.
- How would your decision be altered if you followed a duty-based or consequence-based ethical code?

Consider your answers in light of the discussion below.

If one considers the deontological perspective only it may seem simple to make a decision as Graham is breaking the law and duty states that we cannot allow this to go unchallenged. However, our duty as mental health nurses is to Gwen as well; we must always act in her best interests and she believes that her best interests are to maintain contact with her son despite his behaviour. It is her right (rights-based theory) to expect us to allow her to make bad decisions and live her life in the way she sees fit; however, it is also the right of the public for a person carrying out criminal acts to be punished by law in order to protect others from suffering the same fate. The utilitarian perspective may suggest that it is the outcome creating the greatest good that would be the one to follow and, in this case, it may be that the best course of action would be to report the criminal activity as this protects the largest number of people should Graham not confine his criminal behaviour to his mother. However, if she lost contact with her son as a result of his being criminalised and ended her life in distress, utilitarianism may suggest that reporting his behaviour was not the correct course of action. Considering the biomedical approach means that we must consider Gwen's autonomy; she is perfectly capable of reporting her son's behaviour if it should become intolerable to her and she is allowed to make bad decisions if she makes them in the full knowledge of the potential consequences.

As nurses we must always act in the best interests of our patients. However, in this case would best interests be served better by stopping the financial and physical abuse by reporting him or ensuring she continues to see her son by not rocking the boat? Are you acting non-maleficently if you do not report Graham and allow Gwen to maintain her relationship with him, or are you in fact causing greater harm by allowing him to get away with illegal behaviour?

As you can see there is no simple answer to this situation and, if you were met with this or a similarly challenging ethical situation, it would probably become the discussion of many heated multidisciplinary meetings where the team would thrash out the ethical dilemmas and decide on the most sensible course of action as a consensus. This is more defensible in law than making a decision in isolation.

Dealing with our own prejudices

This discussion leads on to our own values and the role of prejudice in our own practice. The ethical position we assume will be based largely on our own value base and previous experience. While we generally enter the caring professions in order to help others, we carry with us many, often unnamed, preconceptions and prejudices that may affect us during assessment. These can be a help as well as a hindrance. As we saw in Chapter 1, formulating a theory in assessment and then doggedly finding clues to prove ourselves right, as in the case of Lucy's black eye, can lead to incorrect assessment of needs. It is also possible here, though, that using these preconceptions can help us to 'walk in another's shoes'. This can help us imagine how we may feel in an assessment situation, which can make us more sensitive to the feelings and behaviours of the person we have been asked to assess.

Practical challenges to assessment

There are many things that may cause practical difficulties when carrying out assessments. Some of these will be connected to the environment and some to the people you may have to deal with, when carrying out a joint assessment, for example. In Chapter 1 (see pages 11–16) we considered some of the practical elements of assessment and difficulties in meeting the basic requirements for an assessment can pose challenges, such as having no private room in which to carry out an in-depth MH assessment, or deciding whether or not to take notes during an assessment. Here we continue this discussion with some clear practical challenges to carrying out assessment not yet considered.

Patient untruthfulness

People do not always tell the truth and this applies no less in the assessment situation than it does in other aspects of life. There could be various reasons for this and the bottom line is that patients have the right to lie to us should they wish to. Often it is your intuition that will tell you that there is something not quite right about the answers that someone is giving – there may be an incongruity between their behaviour and their spoken word. Consider the following case study.

Case study

Dawn was a 29-year-old woman who had taken an overdose of paracetamol, co-codamol and voltarol. She had been in hospital for over five days due to the amount she had taken and the treatment required. Gemma (the Liaison Nurse) carried out a full psychosocial and risk assessment. Dawn was very defensive from the beginning and was determined not to give anything away. She was an ex-policewoman and was obviously very much in control of herself. She was not aggressive or rude, but was determined to ensure that Gemma did not break down her defences. She answered all questions with excellent eye contact but with no emotion, negative or positive, even when pushed on difficult issues such as her suicidal intent and relationship with her young son. Gemma felt very much that the experience was something Dawn felt she had to endure in order to be discharged – she was aware that she needed to go through the process but was only going to give enough to be sent home.

Gemma's task was to assess Dawn with respect to her mental health, social circumstances and risk, to try to ascertain the likelihood of her repeating self-harm or completing suicide and, following this assessment, to ensure any support she may have required was put in place. Gemma paid great attention to non-verbal cues to assess for risk and mental illness as these often give away intent when verbal assertions deny any.

continued . . .

Intuition is served by watching and assessing these cues, mixed with verbal cues, and the learning and experience already gathered from doing repeated assessments.

Gemma asked repeatedly, in different ways, about her intent and any current suicidal thoughts, future plans etc. However, ultimately, Dawn appeared to be back in 'control' of herself now and, therefore, would be unlikely to self-harm again. One unusual response was that Dawn did not regret the overdose, but that as it had not worked she would not do it again. She appeared to have a somewhat fatalistic view that, if it had been meant to work, it would have done and therefore she was now going to get on with her life and do the best that she could to sort her problems out by other means.

Following assessment Gemma discussed Dawn with the on-call psychiatrist as she was unclear as to her intent but was clear that she had capacity and therefore could make her own decisions, including to potentially end her life. It was difficult to assess the level of risk accurately as Dawn was so difficult to 'read'. She was very clear with her answers to questions regarding her intent and any future plans, and her verbal responses gave no cause for concern. However, Gemma was left with the uncomfortable feeling that Dawn had given the answers she knew were required to facilitate discharge and, therefore, Gemma could not be completely confident about the assessment of risk. Dawn's answers to the questions were closed and she never elaborated on anything. She was discharged back to the care of her GP and offered support from the Samaritans. She refused a formal referral but took the card so that she could contact them if she chose to.

In this case we see that the nurse, Gemma, felt there was the potential for the patient to be lying and, therefore, she took the precaution of discussing the case with the on-call psychiatrist in order to ensure that she had considered the situation fully, thus checking her potential decision with another colleague to help prevent bias and to help deal with the discomfort that she felt at possibly having to allow someone to go home despite potential risks. This is a difficult issue for nurses, and all health professionals, because when there is capacity a person has the right to make bad decisions, including refusal of treatment where it is clear that some would be helpful and even the right to end their own lives (Mental Capacity Act 2005).

Uncooperative behaviour and substance use

There are times when the behaviour of patients can make it difficult to carry out assessments. There will always be a reason for this and it is important to resist the urge to become annoyed with the patient and consider what it could be that underlies the behaviour. Doing this will help us find the likely clue that will allow us to understand the patient a little better, and to form a therapeutic liaison with them in which we can carry out the assessment.

Case study

Gemma is asked to assess a 16-year-old girl who has been admitted to hospital with acute alcohol poisoning. The ward nurses are concerned that she is exhibiting unusual behaviour and wonder if she has mental health

continued . . .

problems. The young girl's mother is insisting that she be present during the assessment and becomes very angry when the ward staff state that it is likely that she will not be allowed to be present. Gemma asks the young girl if she minds her mother being there and the response is a shrug, which Gemma takes to mean she does not mind, so her mother is allowed to be present during assessment. When Gemma asks the young girl questions the responses are mainly given in the form of shrugging and angrily expressed excuses for past behaviours. She makes minimal eye contact and spends the whole assessment curled into a ball with her back to her mother. The assessment is not going well.

Activity 4.5   *Communication*

- Read the case study again. What could Gemma have done differently to overcome the barriers to assessment?
- What would you do in order to continue this assessment in a more profitable way?

Outline answers are provided at the end of the chapter.

This was a challenging assessment, and it would have been complicated further had the young lady remained under the influence of alcohol. With the increasing pressure of beds in many hospitals, patients can be declared medically fit for assessment while they are still clearly under the influence of drugs or alcohol. While they are technically medically fit and require no more treatment for physical complications, they are not psychologically fit in this instance. The use of alcohol and drugs temporarily changes the landscape of people's worlds by affecting their perception; they may be more emotional than they would ordinarily be or view the world as a hopeless place when in drink, while ordinarily they are quite optimistic, happy people. In order to facilitate a comprehensive assessment we need to get as close as we can to the 'usual' state of the individual and, for most people, this is not the state they are in while under the influence of drugs or alcohol. So it is important to wait until a person has sobered up before carrying out our assessment. If he or she begins to experience withdrawal symptoms, this needs to be addressed medically in order for a state of sobriety to be maintained without compromising physical health. A good rule of thumb is to ask yourself if you would be happy for this person to drive away from the department – if the answer is yes, then assessment would be appropriate.

Another difficult behaviour to manage in assessment situations is the person being assessed leaving the interview before you have asked all the questions you wanted to ask. If you get the feeling that this is likely to happen, it is important to ask the most important questions such as risk and mental state early on so you can make a judgement as to the urgency of intervention if required. It is also important to discuss these cases with senior colleagues immediately in case there are other issues that need to be considered, for example information from relatives and so on.

Extreme emotion

When we become highly emotionally aroused, human beings find it harder to act rationally, instead operating from the more primitive – reactive – parts of the brain where the primary aim is to ensure we stay alive. This means that the higher brain functions we normally use, which make us reasonable and intelligent, are compromised temporarily and therefore people who are highly aroused are not easy to work with and impossible to assess clearly. When this occurs the primary objective must be to assist the person to calm down before we attempt to assess him or her.

Scenario

Brian has been referred to you for assessment because he is expressing suicidal thoughts. He is brought in by the police who have him in custody awaiting sentence for a rape conviction. The rape happened 17 years ago and the case has only just come to court. On assessment you find he is extremely angry and cannot answer your questions clearly as he sees you as a representative of the system that has just convicted him of a crime and he does not agree that this conviction is justified. He answers all your questions aggressively; he does not appear to have signs of mental illness but he is quite clear that he will kill himself if he goes to prison. He becomes so angry you begin to feel threatened.

In this situation it is difficult to get a clear picture of the risks and health issues that may be present as it is clouded by the emotion that is present. The first thing to ensure in this situation is your own safety. If you feel at risk, ask another person to be present stating clearly why, or remove yourself from the assessment and try again at a later time. If it is possible to ask the person concerned to use breathing techniques to calm himself, this can be helpful; however, this is most useful when the emotional response is that of sadness or fear, and it would be difficult in this particular situation. In the case of Brian, some information could be gathered from the people who have been around him in custody, as they may be able to tell you if he has reported or exhibited any symptoms of depression or other mental health issues in recent times. Once you have as much information as you can get, it would be important to discuss this case with someone senior as it is likely that, since a custodial sentence is likely, the risk of suicide will remain high. Once a management plan has been agreed, it would be very important to clearly share this with those who will be managing him in custody in order to maximise his safety.

Differing professional opinions

There will always be times, within the multidisciplinary team, when different professionals favour different courses of action, and this can apply to the assessment scenario in the same way as in everyday healthcare. Different individuals have different perspectives; they see risks differently and identify different priorities in the assessment process. Communication can become strained at times like these and it is very important to be clear about your point of view and explain the reasoning behind your suggested course of action. Obviously, negotiation and compromise are watchwords here. Be careful not to lose sight of the patient's needs in the discussions. It can be helpful to explain to the patient the difference of opinion and ask him or her to help make the decision regarding what happens first. If you do this, be aware of the risks that exist in the current situation and be realistic. If one course of action proves ineffective, the next one can then be tried.

Managing risk in assessment

As the assessment process varies in nature, if not in format, for each individual the risks inherent in each assessment may vary. There are some common risks that we can minimise with care and some of them are outlined here.

Verbalised risk

Sometimes patients tell us when they have plans to harm themselves or others, and when this happens we have a duty of care to make sure action is taken to protect those at risk. This includes taking the step of breaking confidentiality, although you should endeavour to try to get the person to agree to sharing the information prior to breaking confidentiality in order to minimise the impact on the therapeutic relationship.

Child protection

Other risks arise when there are children involved. Make sure you outline the boundaries of confidentiality at the beginning of the assessment as this will minimise the shock of, for example, contacting social services when it becomes clear from assessment that there are children at risk. Again, in this situation the requirements of confidentiality are lapsed in favour of protecting any children who are deemed to be vulnerable. This duty of care extends to the whole of UK society, not just the caring professions, via the Children Act 1989.

Personal safety

During the assessment certain steps can be taken to minimise risks to personal safety. Ensure you always have access to an exit and that you are closer to it than the patient at all times. If you feel at risk in an assessment situation make your excuses and leave; you can return with a colleague to support you in completing the assessment. Consider carrying out assessments in pairs where possible as this automatically increases personal safety. Where possible you should also make yourself aware of the risk history of an individual where this is known in advance of the assessment, although there is the argument that this could colour your opinion of the person concerned and could also put you at risk unnecessarily.

Difficult relatives

Relatives and carers of people who are undergoing assessment can sometimes be challenging. Make sure that you are communicating as clearly as possible with them in order to minimise any misunderstanding, and share as much information as you can with permission from the patient. Remembering that these people have information that can be very useful in the assessment process helps us to be respectful of their opinions and to value their views. It is also possible that they will take over the care responsibilities of this person in the future so it is essential that we try to maintain a good working relationship with them.

Prejudicial practice

The importance of self-awareness cannot be overestimated. We have a duty to challenge ourselves and our own practice wherever we note discomfort or difficulty in dealing with patients. We are expected to operate with *unconditional positive regard* to patients without being influenced by their previous actions or behaviours. This is a great challenge and two good rules of thumb to help guide us are to 'do as you would be done by' and to ask ourselves if we would be happy for our closest relatives to receive the care we are providing.

Emotional risk

As human beings, sometimes we have emotional reactions to the stories patients tell us. In this instance supervision and support from managers and mentors become essential in helping us to make sense of the experience and learn from it. Honesty is important here, and letting the patient know that what he or she has said has had a big impact is usually acceptable as the patient may well have noted it anyway. The issue must then be dealt with appropriately in supervision in order that it does not then become a bigger issue and affect your ability to care for that person.

Conclusion

Providing truly person-centred care is a challenge and conducting an assessment, as we have seen, poses many challenges in addition. Sometimes there are confounding issues, such as lack of resources, including time, which make the process even more difficult. Then again there may be communication issues, such as a person being too psychotic to be able to take part successfully in the assessment. Sometimes emotions can get in the way; even our own behaviour can create a barrier to carrying out a successful assessment. There are more potential challenges than can be dealt with in one chapter, so each time you come up against a challenge to assessment it is important to remember that we do not work in silos and to request advice/assistance as required. Reflective practice is one excellent way to learn from our challenges and can provide you with an increasingly robust and flexible toolkit in dealing with future challenges.

> **Chapter summary**
>
> In this chapter we have explored some of the issues that may pose a challenge to the assessment process. We first revisited some of the political, technical and legal issues we encountered in Chapter 1, and then looked in a bit more detail at the economic issues that can challenge our assessments. The social and cultural impact of assessment was considered via a research summary. The chapter then moved on to consider some of the ethical issues that can become a challenge in the assessment process and took a further look at some practical challenges, including talking to people who are highly emotional. We finished this chapter by considering some of the risk issues that may pose a challenge to assessment and will go on to look at ways of managing these when things go wrong in Chapter 7.

Activities: brief outline answers

Activity 4.1: Critical thinking (page 58)

In the NICE guidance document on Anxiety there is no clearly outlined section on assessment issues; however, on reading further you will have noticed that there is guidance on the assessment issues woven into the document, for example 'Ask about relevant information such as personal history' and so on in Step 1. In the BPD guidance there is a more obvious section on assessment issues; however, this is not the only guidance within the document so it is essential that you read the whole thing, as other suggestions are made within it that are important to consider when carrying out assessment, such as communication issues and developing a trusting relationship.

Activity 4.2: Critical thinking (page 59)

Every aspect of *The Code* has an impact on the assessment process.

Activity 4.5: Communication (page 67)

Even well-adjusted adolescents are at a developmental stage where they are unlikely to behave well or answer questions honestly in front of their parents. If there are issues of dysfunctional family life or even abuse, the presence of a parent in an assessment can be catastrophic. Here, Gemma has given in to fear of the mother becoming angry with her and, anxious to avoid a confrontation, she does not carefully check with the young lady that she is comfortable having her mother present during the assessment. This immediately compromises the quality of the assessment, and both Gemma and the patient suffer as a result.

A parent's concern for their child is perfectly understandable and needs to be considered too. Many parents wish to be present in such situations so that they can gain a better understanding of the cause of the problems and offer support and caring to resolve the situation. If Gemma had taken the time to explain to the mother the concerns regarding the complication of adolescent behaviour in front of parents and the need to ensure that the young girl is given every opportunity to respond honestly in confidence, the mother may well have understood this and calmed down enough to allow the assessment to carry on without her. After the assessment, if the young lady was willing, the mother could be brought in to discuss issues that both Gemma and the young lady agreed could be usefully addressed by the mother, allowing her to be involved with her daughter's care and gain a better understanding of the situation. As the mother is already in the assessment scenario, it would be advisable for Gemma to explain to the young lady that she was just going to have a word with the mother outside. Taking the mother aside, Gemma could explain the above and ask her to remain outside for the rest of the assessment, reassuring her that as much information as possible would be shared after the assessment, assuming the young lady agrees.

Further reading

Barker, PJ (2004) *Assessment in Psychiatric and Mental Health Nursing: In search of the whole person.* Cheltenham: Nelson Thornes.

This is a comprehensive book covering the theory of assessment and providing a solid foundation for practice.

Colliety, P and Horton, K (2012) Confidentiality, in Gallagher, A and Hodge, S (eds) *Ethics, Law and Professional Issues: A practice based approach for health professionals.* Basingstoke: Palgrave Macmillan.

This is an interactive chapter that helps you to get to grips with the often difficult issue of confidentiality in practice.

Useful websites

www.justice.gov.uk/protecting-the-vulnerable/mental-capacity-act

This website provides a link to the Mental Capacity Act and the Code of Conduct attached to it.

www.nice.org.uk

Search the NICE website for guidance on all aspects of mental and physical healthcare.

www.nmc-uk.org

The Nursing and Midwifery Council has a wealth of information relating to practice as a professional and student nurse or midwife in the UK, including many free downloads.

Chapter 5
Principles of decision making

Sandra Walker

NMC Standards for Pre-registration Nursing Education

This chapter will address the following competencies:

Domain 1: Professional values

4. All nurses must work in partnership with service users, carers, groups, communities and organisations. They must manage risk, and promote health and well-being while aiming to empower choices that promote self-care and safety.

4.1 **Mental health nurses** must work with people in a way that values, respects and explores the meaning of their individual lived experiences of mental health problems, to provide person-centred and recovery-focused practice.

Domain 2: Communication and interpersonal skills

7. All nurses must maintain accurate, clear and complete records, including the use of electronic formats, using appropriate and plain language.

Domain 3: Nursing practice and decision-making

4. All nurses must ascertain and respond to the physical, social and psychological needs of people, groups and communities. They must then plan, deliver and evaluate safe, competent, person-centred care in partnership with them, paying special attention to changing health needs during different life stages, including progressive illness and death, loss and bereavement.

6.1 **Mental health nurses** must help people experiencing mental health problems to make informed choices about pharmacological and physical treatments, by providing education and information on the benefits and unwanted effects, choices and alternatives. They must support people to identify actions that promote health and help to balance benefits and unwanted effects.

9. All nurses must be able to recognise when a person is at risk and in need of extra support and protection and take reasonable steps to protect them from abuse.

9.1 **Mental health nurses** must use recovery-focused approaches to care in situations that are potentially challenging, such as times of acute distress; when compulsory measures are used; and in forensic mental health settings. They must seek to maximise

continued . . .

service user involvement and therapeutic engagement, using interventions that balance the need for safety with positive risk-taking.

10. All nurses must evaluate their care to improve clinical decision-making, quality and outcomes, using a range of methods, amending the plan of care, where necessary, and communicating changes to others.

NMC Essential Skills Clusters

This chapter will address the following ESCs:

Cluster: Care, compassion and communication

2. People can trust the newly registered graduate nurse to engage in person centred care empowering people to make choices about how their needs are met when they are unable to meet them for themselves.

Cluster: Organisational aspects of care

10. People can trust the newly registered graduate nurse to deliver nursing interventions and evaluate their effectiveness against the agreed assessment and care plan.

Chapter aims

By the end of this chapter you should be able to:

*   apply basic decision-making principles to your own practice;
*   analyse a decision you have made in order to learn from it;
*   understand the complexities of the decision-making process;
*   describe factors that influence errors in practice.

Introduction

Scenario

Every day we make assessments and decisions without conscious thought, such as the decision to sit down.

Assessment information

*   Chair looks sturdy (observation).
*   Chairs usually hold a person's weight (assumption).

continued . . .

- Previously when I have sat on a chair it has not collapsed (pattern-matching previous experience).
- I am tired and need to sit down (personal need).
- The chair is unlikely to collapse if I sit on it (prediction of outcome).

Decision

- I am going to sit down.

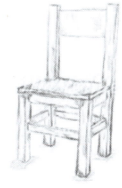

Figure 5.1: Shall I sit down?

In this chapter we consider the basic principles of decision making and explore the complexity of the process via text and exercises. We will look at some theory on decision making and how it applies to mental health practice, and consider certain models that can be useful in helping us to make decisions and explore decisions once made in order to learn from them. We will look at the importance of clinical judgement and the essential element of service user involvement in decisions made. At the end of the chapter we will briefly consider risk in decision making, in particular the principle of positive risk taking.

The assessment process leads naturally to decision making. When looked at in detail decision making is a complex process, but one that often happens very quickly. In Chapter 1 it was noted how we make assessments about many things in the course of a day in order to live effectively. Decision making is part of the same process. We make hundreds of decisions every day, some small, some big, and in each case, in addition to the assessment and assumptions we make, we also have to look to the future and predict what the likely outcome may be. The theory on decision making is vast and it is not possible to cover it in detail here, so some of the most useful information has been chosen to help explore the decision-making process.

What is a good decision?

It is almost impossible to make clinical decisions with perfect outcomes all of the time. Clinical decisions are made from a combination of knowledge of the resources available; the needs and wishes of the patient; the knowledge and experience of the nurse; and knowledge gleaned from literature. There are some decision-making tools that may help fill some of the gaps in the knowledge base, but these should only be used to help make the decision, not make the decision itself. Broadly speaking, in legal terms, it is suggested that a reasonable decision is one that, given the same information and circumstances, a similar person or group of people would have made.

Healthcare is extremely complex and decision making within mental health is likely to be fraught with uncertainty that needs to be addressed as part of the process. Policy drivers and the focus of evidence-based care have increased the scrutiny of decisions made and, where things have gone wrong, the subsequent investigations often take a consequentialist approach, judging the quality of the decision on its outcome (see 'Consequence-based theory' in Chapter 4, page 63). Since this is the case, we can see how important it is to carefully document the decision-making process at the time, so the rationale for that decision can be seen.

It may be becoming clear that it is difficult to define clearly what a good clinical decision is, but in general it is:

> *a decision deemed, in discussion with others (including the patient) and in view of the available information and evidence, to be the one most likely to lead to a positive outcome for the patient.*

Judgement

In healthcare, judgements and decisions are intertwined and there is often no distinction made between the two, although they are really separate entities. A judgement occurs when we assess the alternatives and the decision happens when we choose which one to action.

Case study

James is an informal patient on an acute ward with an acute exacerbation of schizophrenic symptoms. He has been engaging well with his treatment programme and has asked to go on unescorted leave. He has a history of challenging behaviour related to one particular voice, which keeps telling him he is going to be locked up for good. In the past James has gone on unescorted leave and sometimes returned drunk.

Activity 5.1	*Decision making*

- Consider the above case study and decide whether James should go on leave or not.
- When you have made your decision, write your rationale for your decision.

An outline answer is provided at the end of the chapter.

Did you decide to give James leave or not? There would be clear arguments for either decision in this case. Let us explore a little further the potential outcomes of these decisions.

Case study

James approaches Gemma, who is the nurse in charge, and outlines his request for leave. Gemma decides, on carrying out the risk assessment required by the ward, that as he is actively experiencing hallucinations he should remain on the ward. James is disgruntled but reluctantly agrees to stay. Gemma has been qualified for one year and the last patient she approved for unescorted leave did not return and went absent without leave (AWOL), having to be escorted back to the ward by the police.

Later in the day James is found being sick and admits to having taken an overdose of paracetamol in response to distress at the voices telling him this is all part of the plan to keep him locked up. After the event, when the circumstances leading up the overdose were reviewed, it was found that Gemma had only written 'leave refused' in his care record with no clear rationale for the decision being made.

Activity 5.2   *Reflection*

- Looking at the rationale for your decision in Activity 5.1, if it was no, what factors influenced you?
- On reflection, can you think of ways this crisis could have been averted?

Consider your answers in light of the discussion below.

First, it must be noted that had James not overdosed and the day passed uneventfully, the decision would have looked, at face value anyway, as if it were the right one for that situation. As we now know that there were clear risk events following the decision, we can consider some of the factors that would have affected Gemma's decision-making process. These could include her lack of experience, as having been qualified for only one year she did not have a huge bank of previous experience to help her consider the risks inherent in allowing someone off the ward. The fact that her most recent experience with granting leave ended badly made her less willing to take a positive risk for James and she did not discuss her decision with any colleagues in order to help in her thinking process. The decision to refuse leave inadvertently fed into James's hallucination about being locked up, hence reinforcing his fears with regard to this and causing intense distress. Additionally, although Gemma knows how the research shows that patients need to be gainfully occupied when on the ward and that this has a direct correlation with challenging behaviour, she did not consider that in this instance. The fact that she had underreported the decision-making process meant that she would find it very hard to justify her actions should it become necessary to do so in the future.

Case study

In this version of events, Gemma decides that the risks of allowing James leave are less than asking him to remain on the ward in view of his hallucinations. In discussion with him during his risk assessment she asks him how active this voice is and if he has any plans to harm himself or others. He states the voice is not overly intrusive and that he has no plans to harm anyone and he does not intend to drink alcohol during his leave. He appears rational, clearly having capacity and insight into his illness at the time of the assessment, and Gemma asks him to agree to a plan of action should he begin to feel unsafe in the community, which includes ringing the ward so that help can be arranged if he cannot immediately return. She documents this whole conversation and the reasons for her decision to allow leave once she has discussed it with the team on duty and agreed it with them.

While on leave James does go to the pub and gets into a fight with a man who says 'you should be locked up' and the ward gets a call from the ITU later in the day alerting them to what has happened.

Activity 5.3   *Reflection*

- Looking at the rationale for your decision in Activity 5.1, if it was yes, what factors influenced you?
- On reflection, can you think of ways this crisis could have been averted?

Consider your answers in light of the discussion below.

Again it must be said that had James returned from his leave without incident this would have been seen as the correct decision to make, but in light of the unfortunate events that occurred, what may have influenced Gemma's decision-making process here? It seems that, despite her lack of experience, she asked sensible, coherent questions during the risk assessment to ascertain the likelihood of an incident during leave. She is aware from reading about schizophrenia that people manage to live very successfully in the community with active symptoms and knew that it was unlikely that he would be able to remain in hospital until his hallucinations subsided completely due to pressure on beds, so she deemed it sensible to allow a short visit to test out his ability to cope in the community. The same factor that made her say no in the previous case study influenced her to say yes in this one as she was aware that his derogatory voice could be reinforced by insisting that he stay on the ward when he wanted to go out. There is no way that Gemma could have predicted that James would meet a drunken man who would directly feed into his hallucinations while away from the ward. Gemma has also read about the requirements of positive risk taking in helping people to recover and considered that this was an important factor here. She had discussed it with her colleagues in order to draw on their expertise in addition to her own and, having gained their agreement on her proposed plan of action, allowed his leave. The fact that she had documented the whole decision-making process so carefully meant that she was able to defend her decision during the subsequent investigation and the investigating team commended her on being so thorough and believed that they would have made the same decision in her position.

With hindsight, both these situations may have been averted with a compromise, such as allowing leave but sending a member of staff as escort rather than allowing unescorted leave. If the concerns regarding his safety had been carefully explained to him, James may well have been happy to agree to this compromise, thus ensuring that his hallucinations were not intensified either by having to remain on the ward or by meeting a drunken man in the pub.

The level of experience of staff has been shown to have an active influence on the quality of decision making. Staff with more experience are more likely to make decisions that have a positive outcome and are more likely to have a sensible approach to positive risk taking. Some practitioners take a defensive practice approach and this can lead to overly restrictive practices that negatively impact on the patient.

Scenario

Jim is 23 years old and has been recommended to attend a college course that will help him gain his key skills and improve the chances of his being employed in the future. Although he usually lives in the community, he is currently an inpatient on an acute unit following a severe manic episode. The last time he attended college, just prior to admission, he became very agitated and anxious, causing him to run away from the escort who had attended to support him and going missing for two days. He is recovering well on the ward and it is his day to attend college. The multidisciplinary team has agreed with Jim that he should attend college as it is an important part of re-establishing his life in the community and support has been arranged to take him. The nurse on duty is extremely busy and does not believe that the college trip will pass uneventfully; therefore, when Jim tells her that he has not slept well the previous night, she immediately decides that she is sure he would be better off remaining on the ward that day and refuses to allow him his escorted leave to attend college despite his protests.

In this scenario, it could be perfectly reasonable to insist that Jim remain on the unit and not attend college, but here the nurse was guided by her own fear that something might go wrong instead of risk assessing carefully, thinking through possible scenarios and planning for any risky eventuality, so that Jim was able to take advantage of his college course while remaining as safe as possible. So Jim was overly restricted despite the best efforts of the team. The Mental Health Act (Jones, 2009) guiding principles regarding least restriction are best applied here and it is important to note that decisions need to be taken in light of the best interests of the patient, *not* those of the practitioner.

Influencing good decision making

In healthcare we are dealing with people, who are all different and often unpredictable. So how do we make decisions that are likely to have a positive outcome? Remember, even when a decision has an unwelcome outcome that does not necessarily mean that the decision was not the right one at the time. So let us look at the steps we can take to begin to address these difficulties. Being organised is one of the best ways to give yourself space to be able to approach important decision making in a calm, unhurried manner.

Environmental management

First, you can take steps to organise your workday well. Make sure any staff you are responsible for have clear instructions for tasks; reduce interruptions from external sources – for example, only checking emails during certain hours and using protected time for patient interaction; and ensure that there are activities to occupy patients in a ward environment. Such steps are essential in reducing the likelihood of making a poor decision in clinical practice. Time management is also important, as taking the time to consider the options from a professional and patient perspective can save a lot of time in having to explain poor decisions made in haste and dealing with the aftermath, for example increased challenging behaviour.

Overconfidence

It is essential that you actively question yourself when facing important decisions. Overconfidence can be a dangerous quality in healthcare, as the information that occurs to you first when making a decision is not necessarily the best evidence overall. It could be based on recent experience, for example as in Gemma's experience with her previous patient going AWOL when on unescorted leave. So considering all the options increases the likelihood of a correctly made decision. This is further strengthened by discussing the situation with others, as group consensus is stronger than individual decision making.

Evidence-based information

In some cases there are 'base rates' that can help us make a decision. To illustrate, the research around self-harm and suicide suggests that someone with a history of self-harm is at higher risk of suicide than those who have not self-harmed. So it would be important to ask the patient if he or she had any plans in this area when gathering information to inform your decision making. Doing this shows that you actively considered the possibility and can demonstrate, assuming the person says he or she hasn't any intentions, that at the time of assessment and decision making the risk of self-harm or suicide was low. So being well informed about your patient's illness and current condition is essential.

Intuition

'I just knew something was wrong!' Can you think of times in your life when you have either thought this or heard someone else express it? There are many definitions of intuition and much debate about which one is correct, but many agree that the most intuitive nurses are usually the most experienced ones and it may be that this seemingly spontaneous way of operating is actually born of internalised knowledge and experience. Benner (1984) suggests that nurses new to practice will use policies, procedures and tools to help them make decisions, but more experienced nurses rely more on intuition. It follows from this assertion that, if this process is followed, intuition is based on internalised knowledge and is therefore not as ethereal as could be feared. While it would be dangerous to rely solely on intuition, it can provide some useful pointers for generating hypotheses.

Reducing bias

This topic has appeared frequently in this book and again the issue of questioning your instincts is important. Human beings are constantly pattern matching, a technique that is essential for successful living, but in the case of decision making it can represent a real block to good practice. Having stereotypical views of patients is a major block to quality care delivery. We have seen the effects this can have on the assessment process and the effect is no less potent on decision making. It is essential that you understand your own values so you can ensure that these values are then not distorting your decision making. We must be honest with ourselves when these influences are noticed and reflect accordingly.

Decision-making tools

There are many decision-making tools available and it is beyond the scope of this chapter to consider them in detail. The main thing to guard against with any tool is using it to make the decision for you instead of using it as an additional information source that influences the decision-making process. These tools need to be used alongside your clinical judgement, not instead of it. Read the theory below and then take the following case study as an example of how things can go wrong.

Theory

In many emergency departments a tool called the 'Modified SAD PERSONS scale' is used to help identify people attending with self-harm who are at risk of suicide. This tool looks at the 10 risk factors considered most significant for suicidal patients. The patient is asked questions regarding each element and the overall score is calculated, each yes answer scoring 1 point. A score of less than 3 is taken as low risk, 3–6 medium risk and above 6 high risk. The points checked were as follows:

Description	Characteristic
S = Sex	Male
A = Age	<19 or >45 years
D = Depression or hopelessness	Admits to depression or decreased concentration, appetite, sleep, libido

Table 5.1: Modified SAD PERSONS scale (taken from Ryan et al., 1996)

Description	Characteristic
P = Previous attempts/ psychiatric care	Previous inpatient or outpatient psychiatric care
E = Excessive alcohol or drug use	Stigmas of chronic addiction or recent frequent use
R = Rational thinking loss	Organic brain syndrome or psychosis
S = Separated, divorced, or widowed	
O = Organised or serious attempt	Well thought out plan or life-threatening presentation
N = No social support	No close family, friends, job, or active religious affiliation
S = Stated future intent	Determined to repeat event or ambivalent

Table 5.1: Continued

Case study

In one emergency department the instruction was that, if the person scored less than 3, he or she could be considered for discharge without further MH input. Each morning the staff from the MH team would review all the notes of patients who had been admitted with self-harm since the end of the previous shift and as part of this process would check the SAD PERSONS score. On several occasions it was noted that patients had been sent home with a score lower than 3, but the person completing the tool had not noticed that one of the questions answered with a point was 'stated future intent'. Therefore, because the focus was on the number, not the patient's responses, patients at clear risk of suicide had been sent home on several occasions. This then meant that these people had not received the care they probably needed and the MH team had to carry out remedial work to ensure they were followed up in the community, which was not always possible because the contact details were incorrect.

Service user involvement

In order to strengthen the decision-making process and maximise the chances of a positive outcome in clinical care, it is of paramount importance that the service user is involved in the decision-making process. Making decisions on behalf of others when they have the capacity to make their own decisions undermines and devalues them as people and this can have devastating effects on both their self-esteem and the belief in their own ability to have mastery over their own lives. We can actually disable people by helping when they do not need help. This issue is considered in more depth later in the chapter.

Theory of decision making

The most commonly used decision-making process in nursing is the *hypothetico-deductive model* (Thompson and Dowding, 2002), which involves the following.

- **Cue acquisition** – gathering preliminary information about the patient. Some of this can be gathered before actually meeting the person concerned. Information in this category may include baseline data such as gender, age, diagnosis and reported symptoms.
- **Hypothesis generation** – creating an initial theory based on the information gathered.
- **Cue interpretation** – confirming or refuting aspects of the theories generated in the previous stage. So by applying the increasing information you have from talking to the patient, looking at test results and so on, you can begin to interpret the cues you have gathered.
- **Hypothesis evaluation** – evaluating the pros and cons of each hypothesis and maybe deciding on one as being correct, leading to a choice of treatment options or outcomes.

So, information is gathered via the assessment process and then a hypothesis is created and tested out until a point is reached where a decision can be made.

Activity 5.4   *Critical thinking*

Re-read the case study involving Dawn (Chapter 4, pages 65–6). In this case Gemma decided to send her home with follow-up input from the GP and the Samaritans. Using the hypothetico-deductive model outlined above, work through the case study and use it to deduce possible hypotheses for testing.

An outline answer is provided at the end of the chapter.

Practical decision making – risk

Judgements regarding risk are just one of the types of judgements nurses need to make during their practice. *Social judgement theory* builds on the work of Brunswik, who created a 'lens' model that is very useful for examining decisions once made. A view can be reached regarding how good the judgement was by how the information cues have been used. The lines indicating each cue are weighted (illustrated by thickness) to indicate how much significance has been given to each cue. On the left of the figure is the ecological or real situation. A variety of different cues are linked to this and these cues affect the decision made, on the right of the figure, to different degrees, hence the variation in thickness of the lines to indicate this. The problem with applying any social judgement theory to practice is interpretation. Different people will weight the cues differently and hence come to differing conclusions.

Consider Dawn again from Chapter 4 (pages 65–6). Figure 5.2 shows an example of Brunswik's lens (Brunswik, 1943) being used in practice to examine the decision made. Here, Gemma has considered the patient's capacity, indicators of mental ill health, the fact that the patient states she will not try to kill herself again and the apparent fatalistic attitude ('if it had been meant to work it would have done'; 'as it had not worked she would not do it again') as important factors in making the decision to discharge. Less heavily weighted are the 'Adult female, Caucasian, one child' cues, which are more based on the evidence as the research around suicide indicates that these categories mean she is at lower risk than if she was Asian, or indeed if she was male.

Positive risk

In the *10 Essential Shared Capabilities* (DH, 2004), a document aimed at the whole mental health workforce that outlines the essential capabilities required to achieve best practice in education for staff, the Department of Health defines positive risk as:

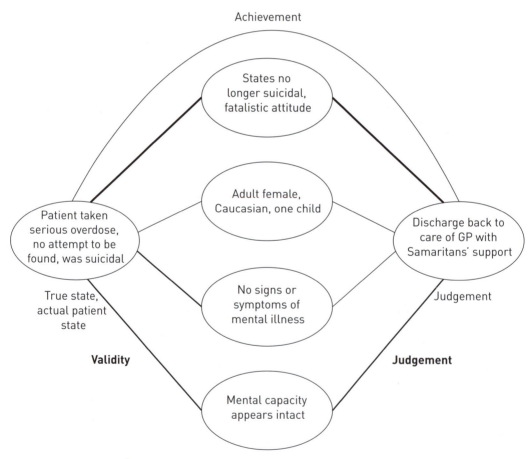

Figure 5.2: An example of Brunswik's lens model in practice.

Source: Based on Thompson and Dowding (2002, p87).

Empowering the person to decide the level of risk they are prepared to take with their health and safety.
This includes working with the tension between promoting safety and positive risk taking, including
assessing and dealing with possible risks for service users, carers, family members, and the wider public.
(p3)

Mental health legislation has long cited the importance of positive risk taking in maximising the chances of full recovery for individuals from mental health problems (DH, 2009). While this is recognised by many organisations, the culture does not yet support the decision making required to enable staff to support patients in this way. This is further complicated by the mixed messages that are received from the Government, namely becoming more cost-effective and promoting positive risk and patient empowerment versus having a zero tolerance approach to socially unacceptable behaviour (Laurance, 2003). This both fuels the fear of litigation from the public should a serious adverse event (SAE) occur and, at the same time, creates an organisation that cannot sustain the level of intervention necessary to avoid such events. Traditional approaches to risk assessment have tended to concentrate largely on historical risk, which, while being valid to a point as history is a good predictor of future behaviour, can result in patients being held back by their past. This can often lead to delayed discharge in the inpatient setting and in a financially restricted climate this is highly disapproved of. This also has associated risks of its own as laid out clearly by the Care Services Improvement Partnership (CSIP, 2007), such as increased risk of aggressive behaviour, promotion of dependence and lowering of staff morale. In support of the need for training and culture change, Smith (2005) points out in his study that, in written feedback, 64 per cent of professionals had indicated they were conservative when considering risk in association with patients who self-harm. As Morgan (2000) points out, we all have to take risks every day and it is unrealistic of services to expect practitioners to be able to eliminate and control risk. However, increased positive risk taking requires more complex clinical skills (Felton and Stacey, 2008) and support from the multidisciplinary team is essential. To support both these aspects, evidence-based practice is of paramount importance (Rosenberg and Donald, 1995), as making sound clinical decisions is difficult in the absence of any formal learning and research to inform practice.

Clinical judgement

Clinical judgement, weighing up clinical information, leads to clinical decision making, choosing between alternatives. In essence it varies little from judgement and decision making anywhere else, but the added responsibility of clinical decision making affecting potentially vulnerable people adds another dimension to it. High-quality nursing care is dependent on good decisions being made and those decisions need to be based on good clinical judgements. The main cue acquisition activity in nursing is the assessment process, and it is the information gleaned here that informs clinical judgement.

Improving clinical judgement

In complex clinical situations the amount of information available to inform a decision can be vast. In order to avoid information overload there are certain techniques we use to shortcut our way through the information and use only the points we consider salient. These techniques, although often useful, can lead to error, so it may help to be aware of these and counter them with some suggested exercises to improved clinical judgement.

Memory

Previous experiences are stored in your memory and accessed when confronting a similar situation. Pattern matching occurs, based on previous outcomes, that tends to make us biased towards one form of judgement over another. These memories are recalled based on how vivid they are, how recently they occurred and how closely they match the current situation. This type of bias can lead to resolute following of one path without proper consideration of the options. In order to combat this tendency, a good strategy is to look for the elements of the situation that don't fit previous occurrences, keeping an open mind and considering reasons why you may be incorrect. Questioning yourself in these ways means the judgement is more likely to be valid and free from bias (see sections on 'Intuition' and 'Reducing bias' above – pages 80–1).

Estimations

In practice, words such as quite, likely, very and highly are often used as descriptors for the amount of something, for example 'He is feeling quite low today.' These words are backed with rating scales that vary from one person to the next so are interpreted in very different ways. This can then mean that people are basing decisions on incomplete information, which can lead to error.

Scenario

Take the example of a mental health nurse, Jo, handing over the care of a patient to the incoming nurse, Jim; as part of the handover information she states that the patient is 'quite low'. This statement gives no reliable sense of how low the patient actually is. In this case, for Jo the word 'quite' means that there is cause for increased concern, whereas for Jim the word 'quite' means noted but not overly concerning. So Jim is at a distinct disadvantage as he has been given substandard information at handover.

Had Jo said something like 'He is quite low today – on a scale of 1–10, 10 being the lowest he has ever felt, he says he's an 8', Jim would have had a much better idea of how low the patient is and how much he should be concerned, and he can make decisions during his working day accordingly. An additional advantage of this approach is that the rating is given from the patient's perspective rather than the personal rating scales of the staff.

Peer review

Peer review is an excellent way of examining decisions made and to critically appraise judgements made in clinical situations. It is also extremely useful in reviewing information and helping move care forward when practitioners are 'stuck' in the care process. Usually done in a group situation, with a facilitator, it needs to be carried out in a context of learning and improving care, being non-punitive and supportive. This technique represents good defensive practice too, as group consensus is acknowledged to be an indicator of good decision making and the judgements made more robust.

Thinking aloud

Where possible, talking through the decision-making process is helpful. This could be done in real time, for example with the team you are on duty with, a supervisor etc. This way others can also examine your judgements and may notice discrepancies you may have missed due to personal bias. This technique helps to collate and synthesise information and, as in peer review, it draws on the knowledge and experience of others enriching the process.

Service user involvement

Patient views and wishes must be upheld wherever possible and the principle of *least restrictive intervention*, as outlined in the Mental Health Act (Jones, 2009), is an excellent guiding principle here. It is important that you maintain excellent documentation that includes decision-making processes and rationales for decisions made, and also discuss the decision with others. If mental capacity is intact, people have the right to make bad decisions as well as wise ones (Her Majesty's Government, 2005). Beales and Platz (2008) state how important it is for patients to be allowed to work in partnership with the care team, as do Leape et al. (2009), who assert that it is essential to have continual input from patients.

Documentation

This chapter would not be complete without a last passing shot about the importance of good record keeping. The NMC (2009) guidelines point out how good record keeping improves accountability and supports effective clinical judgements and decisions. In law, the principle of an action not having taken place if it is not written down still applies, so careful documentation is not optional. Kitson-Reynolds and Rogers (2011) used audit of documentation as an aid to reflection and education around decision making with good effect in midwifery, and Walker (2012) reported how a self-audit tool improved the quality of documentation standards on a low-secure unit.

Self-audit

The following six questions could be used to audit a selection of your record keeping each month in order to ensure that you are practising at a high-quality level. These questions are taken from the NMC (2009) guidelines on good record keeping.

- Are records accurate and written so that the meaning is clear?
- Are records factual and without unnecessary abbreviations, jargon, meaningless phrases or irrelevant speculation?

- Have you recorded details of any assessment and reviews done, providing clear evidence of the care arrangements, including details of information given out about care and treatment?
- Are risks or problems that have been identified and are the actions taken to deal with them shown?
- Have all the colleagues who need to know about the people you are caring for been informed fully and effectively?
- Has the patient/carer where appropriate been involved in the record-keeping process?

Conclusion

It is clear from reading this chapter that the subject of decision making is complex and challenging. It is hoped that there are some practical suggestions here that will help in the process of ensuring that clinical judgement and decision making are as robust as can be expected in an equally complex and challenging clinical arena. As previously stated, good decision making must be demonstrated in clearly documented rationales, working alongside the patient and, in this way, even if the outcome is not as desired, the decision will probably have been the best one made in the situation at the time.

> ### Chapter summary
>
> In this chapter the basic principles of decision making have been considered and the complexity of the process explored. Some of the theory around decision making was considered and how it applies to mental health practice. Ways of helping the decision-making process were looked at and we have explored decisions in order to learn from them. The importance of clinical judgement was considered too, as well as the essential element of service user involvement in decisions made. At the end of the chapter we briefly considered risk in decision making, in particular the principle of positive risk taking.

Activities: brief outline answers

Activity 5.1: Decision making (page 76)

From the case study you may have considered the following in your judgement of the situation:

Pro leave	Against leave
Patient wishes	Acutely unwell
Engaging well	Returned drunk from leave in past
Unescorted leave is part of his treatment	Risk of challenging behaviour
Informal patient	Experiencing hallucinations

Activity 5.4: Critical thinking (page 83)

Cue acquisition – demographic information: female, Caucasian, one child, mixed overdose, no effort to be found, arranged care for the child, serious suicide attempt, wanted to die at the time, defensive, denies current suicidal ideation, no signs of mental illness observed or reported, full mental capacity.

Hypothesis generation –
– still suicidal, wants to get out and kill herself as soon as possible
– still suicidal, masking signs of mental illness
– fatalistic thinking, won't do it again
– embarrassed and ashamed, wants to go home and forget all about it.

Cue interpretation – further questioning regarding suicidal intent, signs and symptoms of mental illness, future plans, relationship with the son and fatalistic thought patterns allow further interpretation of the hypotheses generated.

Hypothesis evaluation – In discussion with senior colleagues the risk of suicide was recognised; however, as Dawn had capacity, other outcomes such as a further assessment under the Mental Health Act would not have changed the eventual decision, only prolonged it, and would have subjected Dawn to unnecessary and possibly distressing additional assessment. All roads led to the action taken so the decision was agreed as actioned.

In this case study Gemma is a very experienced liaison nurse and the colleague who was consulted was an experienced consultant psychiatrist, so they were both happy to take the positive risk required here to allow Dawn to be in control of her life again. A less experienced nurse or doctor may well have opted for further assessment as an inpatient or under the Mental Health Act as a precautionary measure, but both options would have been expensive in terms of cost to the service and to Dawn with the ultimate discharge happening slightly further along the care pathway but with the same outcome.

Further reading

Nursing and Midwifery Council (NMC) (2009) *Record Keeping: Guidance for nurses and midwives.* London: NMC.

This guidance clearly outlines the standards expected for record keeping in all areas of practice, including decision making.

Thompson, C and Dowding, D (2002) *Clinical Decision Making and Judgement in Nursing.* London: Churchill Livingstone.

This is an excellent book that provides an introduction to the academic areas of clinical decision making and judgement.

Useful website

http://sdm.rightcare.nhs.uk

Although there are no shared decision-making tools for mental health available here, this is still a useful resource for looking at the principle of shared decision making in practice.

Chapter 6
Outcomes of assessment
Yvonne Middlewick and Diane Carpenter

NMC Standards for Pre-registration Nursing Education

This chapter will address the following competencies:

Domain 1: Professional values

1. All nurses must practise with confidence according to *The Code: Standards of conduct, performance and ethics for nurses and midwives* (NMC, 2008a), and within other recognised ethical and legal frameworks. They must be able to recognise and address ethical challenges relating to people's choices and decision-making about their care, and act within the law to help them and their families and carers find acceptable solutions.

Domain 2: Communication and interpersonal skills

7. All nurses must maintain accurate, clear and complete records, including the use of electronic formats, using appropriate plain language.

8. All nurses must respect individual rights to confidentiality and keep information secure and confidential in accordance with the law and relevant ethical and regulatory frameworks, taking account of local protocols. They must also actively share personal information with others when the interests of safety and protection override the need for confidentiality.

Domain 3: Nursing practice and decision-making

6.1 **Mental health nurses** must help people experiencing mental health problems to make informed choices about pharmacological and physical treatments, by providing education and information on the benefits, unwanted effects, choices and alternatives. They must support people to identify actions that promote health and help balance benefits and unwanted effects.

8.1 **Mental health nurses** must practise in a way that promotes the self-determination and the expertise of people with mental health problems, using a range of approaches and tools to aid wellness and recovery and enable self-care and self-management.

Domain 4: Leadership, management and team working

6.1 **Mental health nurses** must contribute to the management of mental health care environments by giving priority to actions that enhance people's safety, psychological security and therapeutic outcomes, and by ensuring effective communication, positive risk management and continuity of care across service boundaries.

NMC Essential Skills Clusters

This chapter will address the following ESCs:

Cluster: Care, compassion and communication

2. People can trust the newly registered graduate nurse to engage in person centred care empowering people to make choices about how their needs are met when they are unable to meet them for themselves.

By entry to the register:

11. Uses strategies to manage situations where a person's wishes conflict with nursing interventions necessary for the person's safety.

Cluster: Organisational aspects of care

11. People can trust the newly registered graduate nurse to safeguard children and adults from vulnerable situations and support and protect them from harm.

By entry to the register:

5. Recognises and responds when people are in vulnerable situations and at risk, or in need of support and protection.

Chapter aims

By the end of this chapter you should be able to:

*   begin to understand the complexities of assessment and its various outcomes;
*   consider the legal and ethical implications of assessment outcomes;
*   reflect on the outcomes of assessment when using an evidence-based compared to a locally adapted assessment;
*   define holistic and specific outcomes;
*   explain how mental health nurses can use the outcomes of assessment to be therapeutically beneficial in assisting patients in their recovery journeys.

Introduction

Previous chapters have considered the importance of engaging the patient and carers in the assessment process to ensure that you gain an accurate picture of the patient's issues. You have also had the opportunity to think about different types of assessment. It is, however, likely that the type of assessment that you complete will be steered by the local policies and procedures of the areas in which you are working. This chapter will consider different outcomes that may result from assessments, as well as the complex nature of sharing the information gained and some of the ethical dilemmas this can present.

Confidentiality

The NMC *Code* (2008a) is clear about the need to respect people's confidentiality. It states that:

- *You must respect people's right to confidentiality.*
- *You must ensure that people are informed about how and why information is shared by those who will be providing their care.*
- *You must disclose information if you believe someone may be at risk of harm, in line with the law of the country in which you are practising.*

(p2)

These professional requirements appear to be clear, but do you know which laws can influence this decision-making process? The NMC (2012a) explains that confidentiality is supported by both statute and common law, which includes the European Convention on Human Rights (ECHR, 1950); the Data Protection Act 1998; the Mental Capacity Act 2005; the Freedom of Information Act 2000; and the Computer Misuse Act 1990.

The duty to provide confidentiality also continues after a person's death. There is a 100-year exclusion period for access to medical records and after this period they become available in the public domain (Carpenter, 2013).

Activity 6.1   *Critical thinking*

- Imagine that tomorrow you woke up and found you had a mental health problem that you had not previously had. You have become acutely unwell. Make a list of the people you would want to be given information about your care.
- Would it be obvious to the healthcare professionals caring for you who they could share information with? If not, then how could the staff find out?
- Who is your next of kin or nearest relative? Is this different from the person or persons you would like to have details of your care shared with?

Consider your answers in light of the discussion below.

It may surprise you to know that, despite asking people who come into contact with healthcare services who their next of kin is, there is actually no legal definition in the UK. You can choose anyone as your next of kin as long as you are not subject to the Mental Health Act 1983. The Act has strict criteria relating to the patient's nearest relative, which is the term used instead of next of kin.

According to the Mental Health Act, to be recognised as the nearest relative you must be the patient's husband, wife or civil partner; son or daughter; father or mother; brother or sister; grandparent; grandchild; uncle or aunt; or nephew or niece.

If, however, the patient has been living with someone who is not on the list for at least five years, for example a friend, he or she will be the nearest relative (Barber et al., 2012; Mind, 2013b). The responsibilities of the nearest relative are also clearly laid out within the Mental Health Act. For more detailed information relating to the Act and its application in practice see Barber et al. (2012).

For many people the decision about who to share information with is straightforward; however, consideration always needs to be given to relationships patients may have with the people around them. Patients with mental health problems may have particularly complex histories that may impact on who they would choose as their next of kin or their nearest relative. The relationship between the nearest relative and the patient may also be strained, particularly if an admission to hospital is viewed by the patient as being instigated by the nearest relative.

Activity 6.2   *Reflection*

- Reflect on how it might feel if your nearest relative had been involved in having you admitted to hospital under the Mental Health Act.
- Make a list of what you think your initial feelings towards that person might be.
- Then consider how you might feel once you are discharged. Do you think your feelings would be similar to those listed above?

Consider your answers in light of the discussion below.

At the time of admission to hospital or during the initial involvement of mental health services it is likely that patients may feel angry or upset with their nearest relatives, particularly if patients are unable to recognise that they are unwell. This can be a distressing time for all concerned, therefore it is important that we are sensitive to the needs of all parties. This can be an extremely challenging time and the needs of carers should not be underestimated.

Activity 6.3   *Communication*

- Consider what sort of information you would want if a relative was admitted to hospital or using mental health services. How would you feel if you phoned or visited and were told that, for reasons of confidentiality, you could not be told anything?
- Discuss this with your mentor next time you are in clinical practice and ask him or her how to deal with this situation while maintaining a relationship with significant carers.

Consider your answers in light of the discussion below.

It may be that you are completely accepting of the situation outlined in Activity 6.3, but for many people it can leave them feeling angry and aggressive. If it were your child, parent, sibling or friend, perhaps you would feel the same. It is important to consider that friends and relatives are often more important in the patient's recovery journey than healthcare professionals and therefore need to be treated with respect and dignity (Repper, 2012). It can be a fine balance that can challenge your interpersonal skills. It is important to elicit as much information about who the patient is happy for you to share information with and to ensure that this is revisited as the patient's situation changes. It is not uncommon for the patient to be more comfortable for information to be shared as his or her condition improves. A crisis plan that has been developed by the patient when well can be a useful tool in these situations as it should be clearly stated with whom information can be shared.

Although the NMC (2008a, 2012a) is clear that you need to disclose information if you believe someone is at risk of harm, you need to be aware that you may need to justify your actions to the courts or your professional body (NMC, 2012a). The boundaries can begin to blur once you start to consider in more depth what might be deemed as someone being at risk of harm. Does someone becoming angry and threatening to kill someone actually mean he or she is going to do it? If a patient tells you he or she has had enough and doesn't want to go on, does this indicate a suicide attempt? This is why assessment within mental health is so important, but of equal importance is high-quality record keeping. It is no good working with the patient to complete a comprehensive assessment if you then do not keep an accurate record of what you have observed, discussed and agreed.

Record keeping

> **Activity 6.4** *Communication*
>
> - Make a list of the different methods you use to communicate with your family and friends.
> - Once you have made your list, make a note of how many of these methods you have seen used to communicate about the care needs of the patients you have cared for.
> - How many of the methods you have listed would never be used in relation to patients?
> - Consider the information below about the Data Protection Act 1988 and good record keeping. How does this compare to your experiences of health records?
>
> *Outline answers are provided at the end of the chapter.*

Any records containing information made by, or on behalf of, a health professional in connection with an individual are subject to the Data Protection Act 1988. This includes electronic and written records as well as correspondence to and from other professionals, incident reports, lab reports, emails and text messages (NMC, 2009). As we expand our ability to communicate in different ways it is important to remember that the overarching principle concerns information pertaining to the individual's care regardless of the format. As it becomes easier to communicate in different formats with your friends, colleagues and patients, it is important to ensure that you adhere to all professional and legal frameworks (Data Protection Act 1988; DH, 2007; NMC, 2009, 2011).

The NMC (2009) provides guidance for and the principles of good record keeping. Although all of the points are key to providing high-quality records, points 7, 8 and 9 are particularly relevant to assessment.

7. *You should record details of any assessments and reviews undertaken, and provide clear evidence of the arrangements you have made for future and on-going care. This should also include details of information given about treatment and care.*

8. *Records should identify any risks or problems that have arisen and show the action taken to deal with them.*

9. *You have a duty to communicate fully and effectively with your colleagues, ensuring that they have all the information they need about the people in your care.*

(NMC, 2009, p5)

Any records that you keep should provide a clear audit trail of the patient's assessment and the decisions about treatment that have resulted. This enables the quality of care to be monitored and suggestions for improvements to be made (Burgess, 2011).

The NMC guidance may also help if you are unsure about confidentiality and who in the health-care team should be given information about the patient. If you are unclear about this, it is best to speak with your mentor or another registered nurse in the team, as he or she will be able to advise you and provide any additional support you need. This is why it is important to be clear with your patient that any disclosures that may indicate a risk to themselves or others will be shared with a registered nurse (NMC, 2012a). This also includes situations where a patient asks you to 'keep a secret' for them – it is best to be clear and transparent, no matter how flattering it may seem that the person trusts you. Again, if you feel unsure about this you should discuss it with your practice mentor or your tutor as the sharing of information within the team can build a picture of the patient's current condition.

Scenario

It is extremely busy in the acute admissions ward where you have been working for the last five weeks. Tom has been admitted following a serious suicide attempt. You and your mentor, Sandra, have been trying to assess Tom but he is not very keen to answer any questions. As you go into the office to record the outcomes of the assessment in his electronic records, one of the support workers asks you to take a phone call from Tom's mum. She is extremely worried about Tom and wants to know how he is.

Activity 6.5   *Critical thinking*

After reading the above scenario make a list of:

- what you would do;
- what additional information you might need to help you with your decision making;
- what the legal, professional and ethical requirements are.

Outline answers are provided at the end of the chapter.

Practitioner anxiety following assessment and the legal position

One of the main purposes of assessment is to plan, organise and manage care. This requires decision making that can often lead to anxiety. Have all the bases been covered? Is the person going to receive the care he or she needs? Have all the risk factors been identified and a care package put in place to manage these? Has enough been done to ensure harm-minimisation? These questions may feel familiar – you may have experienced them yourself or, if you are in training, you may anticipate them in the future when you are qualified. The issues identified in these hypothetical questions are important. Assessment should be a collaborative process including the service user (NMC, 2008a) and carer(s), where appropriate, as well as the multidisciplinary team – colleagues from a variety of professional clinical backgrounds. The range of perspectives resulting from such a collaborative approach might appear liable to cause more confusion, but ultimately the discussions that take place should allow a person's problems, needs or risks to be appropriately managed with a clear understanding of who is responsible for providing what. This also ensures collective responsibility for the plan of care and delegation of service and therapeutic provision (Keen, 2009).

At times, as a qualified professional, you may be in a position where you have to make a decision in an urgent situation, but it is very rare that you would not be able to consult with someone else from the care team as well as with the service user and carers where possible. In such circumstances the decision you make is liable to affect a short period of time to cover a crisis situation and you will soon be in a position to consult more widely for a longer-term response to your assessment.

Case study

Sandra is a staff nurse on an acute assessment ward and she had been asked to admit Tom and complete his initial assessment and risk assessment. Tom had recently made a serious suicide attempt and is very low in mood and unresponsive to questioning. Sandra tried to complete the assessment as far as possible, but was a little concerned that Tom would not answer her questions. She recorded her assessment as far as she was able, but ran out of time and at the end of her shift handed over to Diane, asking her to try to find out more and to complete the risk assessment.

Diane got caught up in doing other things and did not complete the risk assessment. Meanwhile, during the early evening, Tom absconded. Thankfully he was eventually found wandering in the grounds and returned to the ward. Diane handed his care over to Yvonne when she started her night duty, but forgot to tell Yvonne that she had not completed the risk assessment.

Yvonne read through Tom's notes and realised his risk assessment had not been done, so she completed it and discovered that he was actively suicidal and was no longer happy to remain in hospital and expressed his intention to leave. As a consequence of her assessment and concerns Yvonne used the nurses' holding power, S.5(4) of the Mental Health Act 1983 (amended 2007), to detain him on the PICU, where he was soon seen by the duty doctor and detained under S.5(2).

It is not uncommon to be concerned that you may not have sufficient information from your assessment to plan care usefully and safely. You can only do your best with the information you have and, where possible, missing information should be sought as soon as is practicable. The law supports professionals so long as they can demonstrate this, which is where record keeping is so important. For instance, if an assessment has been done inadequately (there was little attention given to completing it fully) or not done at all, the outcome from it is likely to be unsatisfactory for the patient at best and unsafe at worst. Under such circumstances the person responsible may also be legally negligent. There are five elements to the tort of negligence: duty of care; breach of duty; harm resulting; harm was foreseeable; and absence of a defence. For more details about clinical negligence, see the website provided by Mind (2013a).

People have a duty of care in three main circumstances: if they are paid to care (while they are in paid employment on duty), if they have started caring (they have to continue until relieved of that duty) and to a blood relative (an old legal element to do with laws of succession). The first two are likely to affect us as health professionals. If a service user is allocated to our care, while we are on duty we have a responsibility to him or her. We also have a duty to that person until we are relieved of that duty. In a ward environment that will be until a suitably qualified person has taken over responsibility of care provision from us. If we are working in a community service there is a responsibility to record our contact with service users and the outcome of our assessments. Any issues of concern must also be handed over to another service if necessary, for example the crisis or out of hours services.

If our planned contact with a patient in our care includes an expectation that we undertake an assessment of some kind, our duty of care will be to undertake that assessment or to hand it over as incomplete if we have been unable to do it for any reason. That way we either fulfil our duty of care or delegate it appropriately.

Activity 6.6   *Critical thinking*

Consider the following questions.

1. In the case study, who had a duty of care for Tom and when?
2. Were either Sandra, Diane or Yvonne in breach of their duty of care to Tom?
3. Did any harm come to Tom as a consequence of a breach of duty of care?
4. If Tom had made a further suicide attempt while he absconded it would certainly have been considered as harm resulting from a breach of duty. Do you think that outcome would have been considered foreseeable?
5. If Tom made a suicide attempt later on while under section and on the PICU, would the situation have been the same?

Outline answers are provided at the end of the chapter.

We can be in breach of our duty of care by commission (doing something we should not have done) or omission (not doing something we should have done). Clearly, if we have done the assessment inadequately (not taken reasonable care to complete it accurately and fully as far as possible) we could be considered in breach of our duty of care by 'commission'. More usually, however, would be a breach of duty by omission – by failing to do the assessment at all.

In order to be found negligent harm has to result from a breach of duty. If a patient suffers no harm the person with duty of care may still have to answer to his or her employers and professional body, but would not be considered negligent in law. If harm results from a breach of duty of care the law will consider whether the resulting harm was foreseeable. If it was then a negligence suit is more likely.

The final element to the tort of negligence is the absence of a defence. 'Necessity' might be considered a defence, for instance if the risk assessment did not occur because the person responsible for doing it was called away to an emergency during which time the harm occurred.

Professional responsibility includes working in a professional, legal and ethical manner. We have just been considering anxieties relating to the outcome of assessments, including the legal consequences of failure to complete an assessment adequately or not to do it at all. Looking after yourself will be considered further in the next chapter, but the focus here is to emphasise the importance of undertaking assessment as thoroughly as possible and to record it appropriately and communicate it to our colleagues in the multiprofessional team responsible for the person's care and treatment.

The ethics of assessment outcomes

In Chapter 4 we considered some of the ethical challenges to assessment. In this section we consider the ethics following the outcomes of assessment. Where possible it is considered good practice to include service users and any carers in the assessment process (NMC, 2008a). Sometimes this results in a collaborative agreement about problems, need or risks, but at other times each may have a very different perspective. Some assessment tools have different formats for service users, clinical staff and carers, for example the Camberwell Assessment of Need (CAN) (Slade et al., 1999). If there is a discrepancy between the differing viewpoints there is a potential for unmet need or risk.

If you assess a service user as being at a particular risk, but the service user does not agree, he or she will be unlikely to engage with the package of care that is put in place to manage that risk. Conversely, if a service user expresses a need that you disagree with and therefore you do not provide a service to address it, the service user is very likely to feel let down by you and the service resulting in disempowerment and potential disengagement.

In Chapter 4 you were introduced to different ethical theories (pages 62–3). From a deontological position there is an ethical as well as a legal duty to the service user. So long as you have acted professionally and diligently it is reasonable to plan care based on the outcome of the assessment, taking into account the rights of the individual to accept or reject care that is offered. From a utilitarian perspective you would need to consider the greatest good for the greatest number and would have to consider how the outcome of the assessment would affect the service user, any carers, family or friends, other service users (where appropriate), other practitioners involved in the person's care and ultimately the National Health Service as far as the cost of care delivery is concerned. From a biomedical framework you would also need to ensure that the autonomy of the service user was respected where possible and that decisions about costs incurred in service delivery were fairly distributed.

A further ethical aspect is linked to resources. It is likely that the outcome of an assessment process will identify a service user's needs. These needs may be quite specialist and there may not be an appropriate service or resource to address them. This can prove challenging in the current financial climate. There is clearly a duty to the service user, but in the absence of a resource you may have assessed that particular need even if it cannot readily be addressed. It would be unethical to identify the need and do nothing. In collaboration with the multidisciplinary team you may find some resource or a similar provision that may help. The minimum requirement would be to document the person's need and the lack of resources and pass the information on to someone more senior, such as your mentor, another registered practitioner or the clinical manager, as they are responsible for enhancing services in line with the requirements of clinical governance (RCN, 2013). Only by identifying a problem can a case of need be created to try to gain resources to meet it (Howatson-Jones, 2012a). For further reading on healthcare ethics, see Beauchamp and Childress (2009).

Signposting and care management

Linked to the previous paragraph, it is important to understand the limits of nurses' responsibility to provide directly for the needs of service users in their care. This, in turn, is related to understanding nurses' role in service user assessment (Howatson-Jones, 2012b). It is equally important that there is an understanding of the role within the wider multiprofessional team, of which other services might be most suitable to meet the needs of the service user. When things go wrong public inquiries identify the likely causes and the learning points from untoward events. A common failure identified is poor communication and collaboration between agencies. In many mental health services health and social care work closely together. In some teams the roles are virtually interchangeable. Indeed, some job advertisements seek mental health professionals from a variety of clinical backgrounds, for example nursing, social work and occupational therapy, to do the same job. While there is a definite overlap in professional roles, there are also elements that are distinct to each professional group. These distinctions are what determines and justifies the particular professions.

A mental health professional may be responsible for overseeing and managing the overall care of a service user. This may include undertaking a therapeutic role themselves, but additionally and sometimes entirely this person will be responsible for signposting – or arranging for the care needs of an individual. The success by which this is achieved relies heavily upon the identified outcomes or results of the assessments that have been undertaken.

In Chapter 2, Activity 2.6 (page 33) asked you to identify all the professionals who were involved in the care of a patient you have nursed. From this you can see that a significant number of professionals may be involved in the assessment of needs and risk. It is essential that the most suitable care is provided for the patient, carers and any dependants by the most appropriate person. This can only occur where assessments and risk assessments have been conducted thoroughly and the outcomes clearly articulated and communicated.

Holistic and specialist outcomes

We have already considered generic holistic assessments that may flag the need for more specific or specialist assessments. Often the latter will have been completed before a service user is referred to a specialist service.

Activity 6.7   *Reflection*

Think about a service user you have worked with during your clinical practice. Choose someone with complex and specialist needs.

- What was the chain of events from the person's initial contact with a health professional (probably a GP) to his or her contact with the mental health services for assessment?
- What was the outcome from that assessment process?
- Reflect on all the professionals who will have assessed the person, when these assessments were likely to have taken place, whether the assessments will have been generic, holistic, specific or specialist, what the outcomes of assessments were in terms of identified problems, needs and risk, and how this influenced the care the person received.

As this activity concerns your own practice, there is no outline answer at the end of the chapter.

Care planning

In order to ensure seamless service delivery and the best quality care for service users it is essential that the identified outcomes of assessment are translated into precise plans of care. This will inform decisions about service provision and implementation of care, which can then be evaluated in due course to establish whether needs have been met and a person's problems and risks managed appropriately.

Activity 6.8   *Critical thinking*

When next in clinical practice identify a service user whose assessment you have been involved with. Ask yourself the follow questions.

- Which assessments were undertaken?
- What were the outcomes/summary of the assessments?
- Do the care plans refer specifically to the assessments?
- Is care being implemented according to the care plans?
- Is care being evaluated regularly?
- Are further assessments being carried out if indicated following evaluation?

As this activity concerns your own practice, there is no outline answer at the end of the chapter.

The nursing process requires all the above elements to be in place and undertaking appropriate assessments and articulating the outcomes from these is the primary and essential stage to ensure relevant care is planned and evaluated.

Conclusion

The outcomes of assessment are complex and will depend on the experiences of the patient. Treating people as individuals and trying to understand their issues from their unique perspectives will help you to engage them in the assessment process. Having an understanding of your patient's viewpoint can help you to deliver individualised care, thus enabling you to make modifications when things don't go as planned. The importance of good record keeping and ensuring that you work within legal, ethical and professional frameworks cannot be over-estimated. Working within these principles will help you in the delivery of high-quality care regardless of the challenges presented.

Chapter summary

In this chapter, we have explained the importance of different outcomes of assessment and considered the legal and ethical implications of outcomes. Beginning with the issues concerning confidentiality, and the concept of 'nearest relative', we went on to examine the sharing of information with others and the importance of complete and accurate record keeping in fulfilling legal and professional obligations. Practitioner anxiety in having to make difficult decisions under pressure was also discussed, as well as the tort of negligence and breaches of the duty of care. The ethics of assessment outcomes were explored from different theoretical perspectives, and the challenge of finding appropriate resources to meet patients' needs was discussed. Finally, the nurse's role in signposting and care management was considered, including referrals to specialist services and the importance of adequate care planning.

Activities: brief outline answers

Activity 6.4: Communication (page 94)

It is impossible to know how extensive your list is. However, many forms of media are now used to communicate with patients, for example texting appointment times and emailing letters. Methods of technological communication are continuously changing and it is difficult to predict how this will progress in the future. Currently the use of social networking is a particularly challenging area and advice about using this is available from the NMC (2012b). Patients may have looked at the internet to gain information about their conditions or treatments. Different forms of media enable us to engage patients in different ways. You must always act professionally, legally and ethically, ensuring you work within the NMC *Code* (2008a). The NHS also provides extensive governance advice outlining a range of legal frameworks that need to be considered (DH, 2007).

Activity 6.5: Critical thinking (page 95)

This will depend on your level of experience. Although you are responsible for your actions you should always check the expectations of your mentor as he or she is accountable for your conduct. If you are a junior student or new to the area, you must always seek help and support from your mentor. If you are more senior and experienced in these situations you may want to gather some additional information.

What does his mum know about the current situation? Gaining an understanding of this can give you a picture of her involvement with Tom when he is at home. It also gives her the opportunity to outline her concerns.

Is she Tom's next of kin? If Tom has identified her as his next of kin it can help you to understand who Tom considers closest to him, although this does not give her the right to information unless Tom consents to this.

If Tom was placed under a section of the Mental Health Act, would she be his nearest relative? Even if Tom's mum is his nearest relative it does not mean that she is entitled to be given information. The Approved Mental Health Professional (AMHP) should make the decision if the nearest relative is to be consulted (Barber et al., 2012; Mind, 2013b). He or she may decide it is 'practicable', thus allowing information to be given, or it is 'not practicable' for some reason, for example if it is likely to cause Tom unnecessary distress (Mind, 2013b).

Activity 6.6: Critical thinking (page 97)

1. All three nurses had a duty of care to Tom, but at different times. Sandra initially had a duty of care for Tom as his care had been delegated to her and she was employed as a nurse. She could not fulfil all of the requirements made of her so handed over his care to Diane. Diane would have assumed a duty of care for Tom because she was employed to care for him and also had relieved Sandra of her duty of care to him, which included the specific duty to complete the risk assessment. Yvonne assumed responsibility for Tom when she came on duty.
2. Although her information was incomplete, Sandra was not in breach of duty by commission (doing the assessment inadequately) because she completed it to the best of her ability with the information available. She did, however, fail to complete the risk assessment and could potentially have been considered in breach of her duty by omission had she not handed over responsibility to Diane.

    Diane omitted to do the risk assessment and was very likely in breach of her duty of care, although we would need more information about her reasons for not completing it. She did not, however, hand this over to Yvonne so left the ward without being relieved of this specific duty. Diane was therefore in breach of her duty by omission.

    Yvonne assumed her duty of care for Tom and fulfilled this by completing the risk assessment. She was not in breach of her duty by commission or omission.
3. Although Tom absconded during Diane's shift he was found and returned to the ward unharmed. Therefore, despite being in breach of her duty of care to Tom by omitting to do the risk assessment and manage the risk, as a consequence Diane would not be found negligent in law. Her manager, employer and professional body may have an opinion on her actions and competence, however.

    Yvonne identified that Tom was a serious risk to himself and managed the risk appropriately by detaining him under the Mental Health Act 1983 (amended 2007) and transferring him to a more secure environment.
4. Given that Tom had been admitted following a serious suicide attempt, harm resulting from his absconding would certainly be considered foreseeable.
5. If Tom made a further suicide attempt on the PICU, it would not be a foreseeable consequence of the earlier omission to complete the risk assessment because Yvonne had rectified that. Questions would be asked, however, about the risk management plan that Yvonne put in place as an outcome of her assessment. Given the seriousness of the identified risk, Tom should have been placed under close observation, making a further attempt very difficult. If this did not occur, Yvonne may well have been in breach of her duty of care and the subsequent harm would be considered foreseeable.

Further reading

Beauchamp, TL and Childress, JF (2009) *Principles of Biomedical Ethics* (6th edn). New York: Oxford University Press.

This book provides additional details about healthcare ethics.

Useful websites

www.mind.org.uk

This website enables you to gain an overview of clinical negligence as well as having lots of other useful information relating to mental health.

www.nmc.org.uk

The NMC provides advice and guidance about many of the aspects covered in this chapter from a nurse's perspective.

Chapter 7
Consequences of assessment
Diane Carpenter, Yvonne Middlewick and Sandra Walker

continued . . .

Domain 4: Leadership, management and team working

6.1 **Mental health nurses** must contribute to the management of mental health care environments by giving priority to actions that enhance people's safety, psychological security and therapeutic outcomes, and by ensuring effective communication, positive risk management and continuity of care across service boundaries.

NMC Essential Skills Clusters

This chapter will address the following ESCs:

Cluster: Care, compassion and communication

3. People can trust the newly registered graduate nurse to respect them as individuals and strive to help them to preserve their dignity at all times.

Cluster: Organisational aspects of care

13. People can trust the newly registered graduate nurse to promote continuity when their care is to be transferred to another service or person.

18. People can trust a newly registered graduate nurse to enhance the safety of service users and identify and actively manage risk and uncertainty in relation to people, the environment, self and others.

Chapter aims

By the end of this chapter you should be able to:

- appreciate the complexities of assessment and the different outcomes that can be the result;
- consider the legal and ethical implications of assessment outcomes;
- reflect on the outcomes of assessment when using an evidenced-based assessment compared to a locally adapted assessment;
- discuss some of the obstacles you may encounter in referring patients on to other areas;
- maintain your own well-being in the assessment process.

Introduction

In this chapter we are going to examine some of the important things to consider after the assessment has been done. The activities will help you consolidate some of the learning you have been doing via this book by considering the issues raised. First, we look at what might happen where things go wrong and assessments don't work out as hoped; we then discuss referring on after assessments and finally examine the most important points to remember in looking after yourself in the assessment process.

Where things go wrong

You would be a rare being indeed if you did not worry about the consequences of assessing patients. Many experienced nurses become anxious from time to time about missing a risk factor or a symptom and what could happen as a result. Consider the following case.

> ### Case study
>
> *May works for the mental health liaison team in the emergency department of the local general hospital, where she assesses people who present following incidents of self-harm or attempted suicide. On one occasion she assessed a middle-aged woman who had overdosed on benzodiazepine tablets. She completed the risk assessment and the woman told her that she was fed up because she had been suffering from back pain for about three months and she wanted the pain to stop. She hadn't wanted to kill herself, but her neighbour had panicked and brought her in for assessment. She felt a little foolish and just wanted to go home. She agreed to go back to her GP for a further assessment of her back condition. Three days later the woman killed herself and May felt awful, believing there must have been something else she could have done and that she must have missed something. Following the news of the tragedy the admission rate also went up because May and her colleagues had lost confidence in their ability to make accurate assessments.*
>
> *There was a local inquiry, which identified that May had completed a risk assessment using her department's risk assessment tool. There was no evidence that she had done this inadequately as every section was completed and fully documented. There was also no reason for May to suspect that the woman required further intervention from specialist services and she had agreed to see her GP, which appeared entirely appropriate.*
>
> *The risk assessment tool, however, was found to have been developed locally and was not a tool that had been tested through rigorous research and found to be valid and reliable. It had not included a section on physical health conditions or family history.*

This story is not unique, but it may also have raised your anxieties. Let us now deconstruct the example and identify the learning points. As the local inquiry had found, May had acted appropriately and was not negligent as she was not in breach of her duty of care, having done everything she should have done. The local assessment tool, although not a published evidence-based tool, had been used for many years without it having been questioned. Just because an assessment tool has not been tested through research does not necessarily mean that it is not valid and reliable. We just do not know whether it is or not. However, chronic pain has been found to be a risk factor for suicide (Hawton and Heeringen, 2000), as has family history of suicide. In this patient's case there was no evidence of a family history for suicide, although it was a particular omission on the form. We have already discussed the evidence base of assessment forms, but it is worth adding here that to include every possible risk factor on an assessment form would make it unwieldy and unusable. Arguably, however, physical health issues should have been included as part of the risk assessment. Following this tragic incident the department adopted a more thorough and evidence-based assessment tool.

The University of Manchester Centre for Mental Health and Risk produces an annual *National Confidential Inquiry into Homicide and Suicide by People with Mental Illness* (NCI), which examines homicide and suicide figures among mental health patients in England, Wales, Scotland and Northern Ireland. Its 2011 summary report for Northern Ireland stated:

> *It is clear that a risk management strategy cannot have much effect in reducing suicides and homicides if it is based mainly on improved care for patients known to be at the highest levels of risk – there are too few of these, according to our sample. Risk management has to be improved for the majority of patients if the few who will otherwise die by suicide or commit a homicide are to be reached. This means comprehensive care plans addressing key clinical problems such as treatment refusal, missed contact and substance misuse.*
> (p9)

It also suggested that risk assessment should not rely only on risk factor checklists, but that detailed history taking can improve the accuracy of risk assessment. The report went on to recommend that:

> *Mental health services should review their risk management processes to ensure that they are based on comprehensive assessment rather than risk factor checklists, and backed up by appropriate skills training and access to experienced colleagues.*
> (pp9–10)

Activity 7.1   *Critical thinking*

Follow the University of Manchester Centre for Mental Health and Risk web link at www.bbmh.manchester.ac.uk/cmhr/ to read the *The Homicide and Suicide Inquiry Report for Northern Ireland* (2011 Summary Report). Identify the most important points for clinical practice, and place these in a logical order. You may also wish to think about the case study above, regarding May, in formulating your ideas.

An outline answer is provided at the end of the chapter.

You will probably have suggested that a detailed client history should inform the assessment process and that the assessment should not rely wholly on checklists, but rather be more comprehensive, and that it should be undertaken by skilled and experienced colleagues. It is likely that you will also have noted that risk management should follow the assessment by developing comprehensive care plans relevant to the patient and including known barriers to care such as problems with engagement and substance misuse.

While you are in training you will be supported in your assessments and risk assessments, and when you are newly qualified you will have a period of preceptorship where this support will continue. Do not imagine, however, that after this you are on your own. It is important to practise within the limits of your competence and it is your professional responsibility to ask for guidance and support where necessary. Preceptorship and supervision are mentioned further on in this chapter.

In Chapter 6 we considered negligence (see pages 97–8) and it would be useful to revise that here to ensure you are familiar with the concepts. The law will support you so long as you acted responsibly and professionally and did all that could reasonably be expected of a nurse with the same level of training and experience. The *Inquiry into Suicide and Homicide* report emphasised not relying wholly on checklists and this is where our professional responsibility for keeping up to date is important. As we have already discussed, it would be impossible to have an all-embracing risk-assessment form that covers every eventuality; but if, as nurses, we keep abreast of the research relevant to our field of practice, we may be able to supplement the questions we ask patients as standard with those based on the most recent and relevant research. The example given was of a risk scenario, but this holds equally for any assessment, whether it is to identify a problem, need or risk.

Assessment across the age continuum

Children and young people

Children's and young people's mental health is more complex to assess than that of adults. A child with depression is not likely to present with the classic symptoms we associate with working-age or older people. Their depression may, for instance, manifest itself in unruly behaviour at school or school refusal. It is estimated that 1 in 200 children under 12 years of age and 2 to 3 in every 100 teenagers experience depression (NICE, 2009), which is a considerable number, and quite possibly underreported. Many teenagers are reluctant to seek professional help for depression because of the stigmas associated with it; at a time when peer acceptance is paramount, appearing out of the ordinary is something that most young people will actively seek to avoid. Similarly, parents may be reluctant to acknowledge that their child has a mental health problem. They are likely to fear the consequences of having their child assessed.

Activity 7.2   *Critical thinking*

Reflect on the paragraph above and, making a copy of the table below, list any further reasons you feel might account for children, young people and parents not seeking mental health assessment and treatment for the child or young person.

	Children	Young people	Parents
Reasons for not seeking mental health assessment	_____	_____	_____
	_____	_____	_____
	_____	_____	_____
	_____	_____	_____
	_____	_____	_____
	_____	_____	_____

An outline answer is provided at the end of the chapter.

The list is almost endless, but illustrates some of the complexities and possible consequences of assessing children and young people for mental health problems. Another factor is the difficulty of assessing younger children who may not have the vocabulary to articulate their feelings. It is fairly common for young children, in assessment, to draw or paint how they feel, but it takes specialist expertise to work with the child to assess them using such media.

Further complexities include the difficulty of observing symptoms. This may be particularly significant in the event of young people with eating disorders or who self-harm, or with children and young people who are being physically and sexually abused. In such cases it is often teachers who may notice symptoms, particularly if a child is reluctant to undress for physical education (PE) or sports. The complexity here is in ascertaining the facts to raise concerns for an investigation, or in broaching the subject with a child or young person. Many young people avoid PE for a variety of reasons and it can be a normal part of adolescence for young people to feel uncomfortable with their changing body shapes. However, all schools and colleges have safe-guarding and child protection policies to guide practice. The Royal College of Nursing (RCN, 2009) reinforces the position for all nurses:

> *Practitioners have an absolute duty to share any concerns they may have that concern possible abuse. Remember that referral is an obligation, not an option.*

You may have had an opportunity for a Child and Adolescent Mental Health Service (CAMHS) placement during your training. If you have you will know that the CAMHS service includes practitioners from a variety of professional backgrounds who work collectively to assess children and young people. If you choose to work in such a service you will be involved in specialist assessments and will become skilled and competent in time.

In adult services, however, you are also likely to meet patients with children and your observation about the mental health of these children is paramount. A mentally ill parent is a significant stressor for a child or young person, who may also be suffering mental ill health or be at risk of becoming mentally unwell as a consequence. Should you have concerns you can discuss these with colleagues from the multidisciplinary team in which you work and/or the GP and other primary care practitioners, such as the child's health visitor, where appropriate.

Older people

Older people require skilful assessment as they may present with complex multiple pathologies relating to both mental and physical health. This means that, for older people, there is not generally one assessment that will cover everything.

Case study

Jane, a mental health nurse, has been assessing Mrs Smith, 78, for depression. Her husband died two years ago following a long fight against cancer. She cared for him until he died. She has two children with whom she has a good relationship, although they live some distance away and work full time. Following the death of her husband she went with her close friend to learn to play bridge, which she enjoyed. This led to a busy

continued . . .

social life. Over the last six weeks Mrs Smith has been unable to get out and about as much. She says she is feeling tired all the time, is not sleeping well and wakes with episodes of breathlessness. Although she sees her friend she has not played bridge for the last three weeks. Mrs Smith tells you that since all of this started she has noticed that her ankles keep swelling, which she believes is due to 'sitting around', and she is having trouble remembering things such as ringing her daughter at the agreed time. This is worrying her as her husband's brother had dementia and she doesn't want to worry her children.

Activity 7.3	*Critical thinking*

Make a list of the mental health and physical health issues you think might be affecting Mrs Smith.

An outline answer is provided at end of chapter.

You may have provided an extensive list. When you are assessing an older person this may be one of the first opportunities there has been to gain a full assessment, possibly due to him or her not having accessed services previously. There are many physical health problems that can manifest themselves as mental health problems in older people, so it is important to ensure a full physical assessment before diagnosing a mental health problem (Nash, 2010).

You can imagine the devastating effects it can have on a patient and his or her family to receive a diagnosis such as dementia for something that could potentially be treated, thus resulting in no mental health problems at all.

The other issue that may be extremely complex is the social situation of patients, particularly if they are unable to care for themselves if they have become frail. As a nurse you need to work collaboratively with patients and their significant others, including carers, to provide support. It is important to remember that sometimes patients make decisions that may be at odds with the wishes of professionals advising them. Healthcare professionals need to respect this and help to minimise risk wherever possible.

Referring on

After your assessment you may need to refer the person on to further services. There are some issues you need to consider at this stage. We have previously discussed in Chapter 1 the importance of having a comprehensive knowledge of the services in your local area, as it is difficult to know where to refer your patients to if you do not know (see 'Resources available to the service user', pages 14–15). Because of the increasingly fragmented nature of mental health services, patients can face a complex array of providers even within the care for one condition. It should always be our aim to minimise the potentially negative impact these service boundaries can have on patients themselves.

Networks

If there is a service you are likely to be referring patients to repeatedly, it would be worth visiting this area to meet key professionals in the team. There are two good reasons for this. First, it ensures you are really clear about the resources offered by the service so you can make sure your referrals are always appropriate. Second, referrals are more likely to go smoothly if you have some sort of relationship with those who work in the service; if they know that you fully understand their referral criteria they will be less questioning of any referral that you make. This type of professional networking helps to minimise the effect of interprofessional boundaries and smoothes your patients' journeys to receiving the care they need.

Information sharing

In some cases, the processes we have to use in our practice can work against us. An example of this is where a service crosses boundaries between counties; consider the following scenario.

Scenario

Imagine you are working in a mental health liaison team based in a large district hospital that provides care for people from two large geographical areas. The patients in these areas are serviced by five different healthcare Trusts, two of which are mental health providers and multiple social care providers. Your liaison team is only allowed to access the electronic records for patients of the service they are employed by, therefore patients attending from neighbouring Trusts with mental health issues are often missing vital information, most notably around risk. The only way you can gather this information is by telephoning the service provider in the patient's locality and this information is often withheld, even then, because of fears regarding confidentiality and lack of a clear service-level agreement about information sharing.

Activity 7.4 — *Critical thinking*

Read the scenario again and make a list of the ways in which this situation may impact on patient care.

Consider your answer in light of the discussion below.

In the situation that exists in this hospital, it is likely that a large amount of time will be spent gathering information that should have been available to read at a few clicks of the mouse: time explaining who you are, why you are calling and justifying your need to know regarding the patient. This all adds to the time you spend undertaking each assessment and reduces efficiency. It is likely that each patient will have to undergo repeated assessments in order for you to gather the information required if the host service will not tell you what you need to know. Difficulties persuading a service to give you information can lead to friction when you are trying to then re-refer the patient to the same service for follow-up care. Management of risk is compromised if you are unable to discover any risk indicators present for patients prior to assessment; important issues can be missed as many patients may not tell you that they are considered a risk. This puts both professionals and patients at risk as vital information could be missing. Inevitably this situation causes a reduction in the quality of the service offered to patients and increases the effect of interprofessional boundaries on patient care. The increasing disaggregation of services that is occurring in healthcare currently often leads to separate parts of a system failing to work together (Harle et al., 2010). This is at odds with the patient-centred, holistic care we are expected to provide and that patients report they prefer (DH, 2004).

Advocacy

This is an essential part of your role as a mental health nurse. Experiencing mental ill health is fundamentally disempowering and the patient voice has often been lost in the provision of care for individuals. Advocating for the patient is key to providing service user-centred care. The belief that someone who is unable to speak for themselves should be supported to express what he or she needs is fundamental to advocacy. Mind (2007) describes advocacy as the process of supporting and enabling people to:

- express their views and concerns;
- access information and services;
- defend and promote their rights and responsibilities;
- explore choices and options.

As a student and burgeoning mental health nurse you will not be advocating all the time, but you must be prepared to fight for the rights of your patients and this skill is becoming increasingly necessary as the boundaries between services increase and resources shrink in the economic climate we are all now facing.

Looking after yourself

As a mental health nurse you will spend a significant amount of time working with people suffering varying levels of distress for a multitude of reasons. Once you start assessing people and enabling them to engage effectively with the assessment process they may disclose complex and horrific histories. This may arouse many feelings in you as the assessor, so it is important that you are able to recognise these and seek appropriate help and support. The emotional nature of patient disclosures may also result in the re-emergence of past feelings if you yourself have had to deal with any trauma. The NMC (2010b) states that pre-registration education should prepare students to look after their own mental health as well as the mental health of others. The Chief Nursing Officer has recommended that regular clinical supervision should be used as part of the support system to help mental health nurses recognise stressful situations (DH, 2006).

- Make a list of all of the support systems available to you, both formal (e.g. via your mentor) and informal (e.g. via friends).
- Once you have done this, reflect on the pros and cons of each.

Consider your answers in light of the discussion below.

Informal systems

Friends and family may have come up on your list as an informal support system. One of the benefits is that they are likely to know you very well and may be able to give you the emotional support that you need. This may enable you to think about issues and consider what you may do differently, with your informal support systems being able to offer you advice because of their knowledge of you. This informal type of reflection may also contribute to how you develop as a practitioner, with friends and family offering an honest opinion in relation to you. It is, however, worth considering the potential for (understandable) positive bias in wanting to support you without having a full understanding of the dilemmas you may be facing.

On a professional level one of the major disadvantages of informal support systems is that you have to be so careful with regard to confidentiality (NMC, 2008a, 2011, 2012a). Another disadvantage may be that your friends and family don't understand how you feel, particularly if they have never worked in this field of practice. If they do not really understand what you do, you may find that they unduly stigmatise your patient group and are influenced by the media. Therefore, their advice and support may be biased not only towards you but also against your patients, which will not necessarily help you enhance your skills and development.

There are therefore many advantages to being able to use effectively the support systems provided in the healthcare organisations where you are placed and within your university.

Formal systems

Reflective practice

Nurses commonly cite reflection as a tool used to develop their practice, but perhaps you have not considered this as a tool to offer you support. The requirement to reflect on practice is embedded in nurse education (NMC, 2010b) and often leads to a number of academic pieces of work dedicated to developing this important skill. Driscoll (2007) suggests that using reflection as an assessed piece of work may cause anxiety about the process, leading to superficial engagement with reflection as a learning opportunity once students become registered nurses. One benefit of reflecting as a registered practitioner is that you generally have more control over what you reflect on; also, the skills developed through academic reflective writing offer a potential learning opportunity by enabling you to explore the literature related to the subject. Howatson-Jones (2010, p6) suggests that *reflection is a way of examining your experience in order to look for the possibility of other explanations and alternative approaches to doing things.* This can help you meet your professional requirement to provide high-quality patient care using best practice or the best available evidence (NMC, 2008a).

There are numerous reflective models and frameworks to help develop your skills in this area and it is important to find one that suits your personal style. Some reflections may be extremely detailed, particularly if they are for an academic assignment, which will encourage you to look at the underpinning evidence. At other times reflection may be less formal, such as pondering while travelling to and from work, or while talking with colleagues. In these cases your analysis may be limited to the experiences of others (anecdotal evidence); this is valuable but may not necessarily include the best available evidence.

One of the benefits of reflective practice is that it can be an opportunity to look inside yourself and it can therefore be done on your own (Johns, 1996) or as part of a group and, unlike clinical supervision, there is no requirement to be with a more experienced practitioner. Consider which is the best forum for you; if you have been involved in a challenging assessment it may be better to reflect with someone who has some experience, or you may be able to reflect on your own and consider how you will improve your practice next time, or indeed what went particularly well. There can be a tendency to focus only on the negative, but there are times when things go unexpectedly well and by reflecting on these you can also further develop your practice.

Case study

Penny was trying to complete an assessment on a male patient who clearly did not want to answer a single question. Once she realised this was going to be fruitless Penny decided to change her tactics, so she put away all the paperwork and asked him to tell her about himself. Although initially he didn't think Penny really wanted to know anything, with a bit of coaxing his story began to flow. By the end of her shift she knew a great deal about him, his family and his experiences. This was a pivotal moment in Penny's career when she realised that, even though she had thought she was person-centred in approach, she had not been. Penny had been really focused on getting the paperwork completed.

If you look at the wording in the first couple of sentences, the language itself does not suggest a person-centred collaborative approach: for example, 'an assessment *on*' rather than 'an assessment with' and even 'Penny decided to *change her tactics*', perhaps suggesting a degree of manipulation.

Penny reflected on this situation and wrote it up for her portfolio so that she could remind herself that one interaction and reflecting on practice can lead to increased self-awareness and the development of professional practice.

Clinical supervision

It is possible that clinical supervision featured on your list from Activity 7.5. Bush (2005, p38) describes it as providing a *nurturing and supportive service for nurses, helping them to reflect critically on their actions or possible inactions in the provision of patient care.* Driscoll (2007) explains that clinical supervision is a form of professional conversation that enables development rather than offering advice.

It is not possible to know everything there is to know about caring for people even when you have been registered for years. The aim of clinical supervision is to develop knowledge and competence through dialogue with other practising professionals to enable a process of learning to improve the quality of patient care (NHS Executive, 1993; Bush, 2005; DH, 2006; Driscoll, 2007).

Mental health organisations have been quite forward thinking in the implementation of clinical supervision. It has occurred in some practice areas since the 1990s. Many mental health areas have established clinical supervision protocols outlining the expectations for its frequency. It is often expected that staff will undertake clinical supervision every four to six weeks. This may also include the requirement to keep records so that improvements in practice can be demonstrated.

Activity 7.6   *Team working*

In your practice area, find out if there are any requirements for the staff to have clinical supervision. Is there a policy outlining the requirements? If so, have a look at it and consider if it outlines a supportive mechanism to improve patient care and if the requirements of staff, managers and the organisation are clearly articulated.

As this activity concerns your own practice, there is no outline answer at the end of the chapter.

One of the criticisms of clinical supervision is that it can sometimes be viewed as a form of management control (Bush, 2005), especially by people whose manager provides supervision. But the main reason for clinical supervision is to improve patient care. You should therefore be able to choose your supervisor, someone you feel will help you but who can also constructively challenge you to develop your clinical practice.

Mentors, preceptors and academic support

While in clinical practice as a student nurse you will be allocated a mentor to support you. This is mandatory and your mentor will have completed an approved mentor training programme (NMC, 2008b). You may also gain support from other members of the clinical team. This can be useful in helping you develop different strategies, as people often work in different ways with patients and you can learn from them.

Once you are a registered nurse you may be offered a period of preceptorship. Although this is not currently a mandatory requirement, many newly registered nurses find it helpful to have a preceptor to support them with the transition from student to accountable practitioner (DH, 2010b; NMC, 2010a; Willis Commission, 2012). When you are looking for your first job it is useful to ask if the organisation has a preceptorship programme, as this is an additional opportunity to gain support.

You should also remember that your tutor might be able to offer you support, particularly if you have had a challenging incident during your placement. Although discussing issues with the clinical team is often the most appropriate thing to do, there may be times when you do need additional support or if your concerns relate to the clinical team. If you are unsure about what to do, you should always speak to your tutor who can advise you.

As more services are reconfigured only the most unwell people will be treated in inpatient services. This leaves many people who have varying degrees of problems in the community and, although this is felt to be much better for patients and their families, it can leave nurses feeling a great deal of responsibility. It is therefore important to ensure that you gain appropriate support to help you develop your practice and enable you to look after yourself.

Conclusion

Assessment is a complex process, fraught with difficulties, and, having worked your way through this book, you are now in a much better position to combat these difficulties successfully. The assessment process provides us with the privileged position of spending time with patients, time that can have an immeasurably important positive impact just by the very nature of the listening role we adopt in gathering the information contained in patients' stories. By keeping patients at the core of the care we provide, remaining well aware of their needs and involving them as much as possible in the process, we will ensure that high-quality assessment is guaranteed in our practice.

Chapter summary

In this chapter we have considered some of the important things required after the assessment has been done. We looked at what might happen where things go wrong and assessments don't work out as hoped. We then discussed referrals after the assessment and considered the most important points in looking after yourself in the assessment process. We have clearly demonstrated the complexities of assessment and the different outcomes that can be the result, while considering some of the legal and ethical implications of these. We have also reflected on the outcomes of using an evidenced-based assessment compared to a locally adapted version and have considered some of the difficulties inherent in the complex healthcare systems we are currently operating in.

Activities: brief outline answers

Activity 7.1: Critical thinking (page 107)

The most important points for clinical practice are:

- a detailed client history;
- a risk management plan;
- comprehensive care plans.

Activity 7.2: Critical thinking (page 108)

You may have considered factors such as:

- ignorance or unawareness of mental health problems;
- not recognising symptoms;
- not associating behaviours with mental health problems;
- fear about being given a diagnosis and its prognosis.
- the consequences of having a mental health problem, including treatment, effects on current and future lifestyle such as employability and social/peer acceptance, and whether inpatient treatment may be required and the disruption this can cause to schooling;
- parents may fear that their child will be 'labelled' as mentally ill at such a young age;
- parents may also hope that, if left alone, the problem will disappear of its own accord and may just be 'normal behaviour' for teenagers, for example;
- parents may feel they are betraying their child by seeking professional help.

Activity 7.3: Critical thinking (page 110)

Mrs Smith may be affected by:

- mental health issues: depression, anxiety and dementia;
- physical health issues: delirium, heart failure or another cardiac issue, hypothyroid, dehydration, diabetes or infection. These are just a few of the many physical health problems that can affect our clients regardless of age.

Further reading

National Child and Adolescent Mental Health Services (CAMHS) Support Service (2011) *Self-harm in Children and Young People Handbook.* Available online at www.chimat.org.uk/resource/item.aspx?RID=105602.

CAMHS has designed this handbook to help nurses and other professionals better understand the issues behind self-harm in children and young people.

Useful websites

www.bbmh.manchester.ac.uk/cmhr

The University of Manchester Centre for Mental Health and Risk provides links to its *National Confidential Inquiry into Suicide and Homicide by People with Mental Illness*, from various years.

www.chimat.org.uk

As well at the CAMHS handbook mentioned in 'Further reading', ChiMat provides information for professionals involved in working with children and young people – follow the other links for more information on mental health and psychological well-being.

www.mind.org.uk/mental_health_a-z/8040_advocacy_in_mental_health

This webpage provides some useful information about the concept of advocacy.

References

Aggleton, P and Chalmers, H (2000) *Nursing Models and Nursing Practice* (2nd edn). Basingstoke: Palgrave.

Aitken, P (2007) *Mental Health Policy Implementation Guide: Liaison psychiatry and psychological medicine in the general hospital*. London: Royal College of Psychiatrists.

Bach, S and Grant, A (2009) *Communication and Interpersonal Skills for Nurses*. Exeter: Learning Matters.

Barber, P, Brown, R and Martin, D (2012) *Mental Health Law in England and Wales: A guide for mental health professionals* (2nd edn). London: Learning Matters.

Barker, PJ (2004) *Assessment in Psychiatric and Mental Health Nursing: In search of the whole person* (2nd edn). Cheltenham: Nelson Thornes.

Barker, PJ (2009) *Psychiatric and Mental Health Nursing: The craft of caring* (2nd edn). London: Hodder Arnold.

Beales, A and Platz, G (2008) Working in partnership, in Stickley, T and Basset, T (eds) *Learning About Mental Health Practice*. Chichester: Wiley.

Bear, MF, Connors, BW and Paradiso, MA (2007) *Neuroscience: Exploring the brain* (3rd edn). London: Lippincott Williams & Wilkins.

Beauchamp, TL and Childress, JF (2001) *Principles of Biomedical Ethics*. London: Oxford University Press.

Beauchamp, TL and Childress, JF (2009) *Principles of Biomedical Ethics* (6th edn). New York: Oxford University Press.

Beck, AT, Steer, A and Brown, GK (1996) *Beck Depression Inventory-II*. Orlando, FL: Harcourt, Brace and Company.

Benner P (1984) *From Novice to Expert: Excellence and power in clinical nursing practice*. Menlo Park, CA: Addison-Wesley.

Bowling, A (2001) *Measuring Disease* (2nd edn). Buckingham: Open University Press.

Brown, J (2012) The therapeutic use of self, in Tee, S, Brown, J and Carpenter, D (eds) *Handbook of Mental Health Nursing*. London: Hodder Arnold.

Brunswik, E (1943) Organismic achievement and environment probability. *Psychological Review*, 50: 255–72.

Burgess, R (ed.) (2011) *New Principles of Best Practice in Clinical Audit* (2nd edn). Abingdon: Radcliffe.

Bush, T (2005) Overcoming the barriers to effective clincial supervision. *Nursing Times*, 101(2): 38–41.

Care Services Improvement Partnership (CSIP) (2007) *A Positive Outlook: A good practice toolkit to improve discharge from in patient mental health care*. London: National Institute for Mental Health in England.

Carpenter, D (2013) Using historical literature, in Glasper, EA and Rees, C (eds) *How to Write your Nursing Dissertation*. Chichester: Wiley-Blackwell. Available online at http://bcs.wiley.com/he-bcs/Books?action=mininav&bcsId=7474&itemId=1118410718&assetId=294078&resourceId=29071&newwindow=true (accessed 14 February 2013).

Cox, JL, Holden, JM and Sagovsky, R (1987) Detection of postnatal depression: development of the 10-item Edinburgh Postnatal Depression Scale. *British Journal of Psychiatry*, 150: 782–6.

Deegan, P (1996) Recovery as a journey of the heart. *Psychiatric Rehabilitation Journal*, 19(3): 91–7.

Department of Health (DH) (2004) *10 Essential Shared Capabilities*. London: Department of Health.

Department of Health (DH) (2006) *From Values to Action: The Chief Nursing Officer's review of mental health nursing*. London: Department of Health.

Department of Health (DH) (2007) *NHS Information Governance: Guidance on legal and professional obligations*. London: Department of Health.

Department of Health (DH) (2009*) Good Practice Guidance on the Assessment and Management of Risk in Mental Health and Learning Disability Services*. London: Department of Health.

Department of Health (DH) (2010a) *Equity and Excellence: Liberating the NHS*. London: The Stationery Office.

Department of Health (DH) (2010b) *Preceptorship Framework for Newly Registered Nurses, Midwives and Allied Health Professionals*. London: Department of Health.

Department of Health (DH) (2011a) *No Health without Mental Health*. London: Department of Health.

Department of Health (DH) (2011b) *The Operating Framework for the NHS in England 2012–13*. London: The Stationery Office.

Driscoll, J (2007) *Practising Clinical Supervision: A reflective approach for healthcare professionals* (2nd edn). Edinburgh: Baillière Tindall Elsevier.

Ensel, WM and Woelfel, J (1986) Measuring the instrumental and expressive functions of social support, in Lin, N, Dean, A and Ensel, W (eds) *Social Support, Life Events and Depression*. New York: Academic Press.

European Court of Human Rights (ECHR) (1950) *European Convention on Human Rights*. Available online at www.echr.coe.int/Documents/Convention_ENG.pdf (accessed 25 January 2013).

Felton, A and Stacey, G (2008) Positive risk taking: a framework for practice, in Stickley, T and Basset, T (eds) *Learning about Mental Health Practice* (pp195–212). Chichester: Wiley.

Francis, R (2013) *Report of the Mid-Staffordshire NHS Trust Public Inquiry*. London: Crown Copyright.

Fredriksson, L and Lindström, UA (2002) Caring conversations: psychiatric patients' narratives about suffering. *Journal of Advanced Nursing*, 40(4): 396–404.

Goldberg, D and Williams, P (1988) *General Health Questionnaire (GHQ)*. Windsor: NFER-Nelson.

Griffith, R and Tengnah, C (2010) *Law and Professional Issues in Nursing*. Exeter: Learning Matters.

Hamilton, M (1969) Diagnosis and rating of anxiety. *British Journal of Psychiatry*, Special issue, 3: 76–9.

Hammond, GS and Aoki, TT (1992) Measurement of health status in diabetic patients. *Diabetes Care*, 15: 469–77.

Harle, T, Page, M and Ahmad, Y (2010) Organisational issues, in Pollard, K, Thomas, J and Miers, M (eds) *Understanding Interprofessional Working in Health and Social Care* (pp138–55). Basingstoke: Palgrave.

Hawton, K and Heeringen, KV (2000) *The International Handbook of Suicide and Attempted Suicide*. New York: Wiley.

Her Majesty's Government (2005) Mental Capacity Act. London. Available online at www.legislation. gov.uk/ukpga/2005/9/pdfs/ukpga_20050009_en.pdf (accessed 6 August 2013).

Heron, J (2001) *Helping the Client: A creative practical guide* (5th edn). London: Sage.

Howatson-Jones, L (2010) *Reflective Practice in Nursing*. Exeter: Learning Matters.

Howatson-Jones, L (2012a) Ethical aspects of patient assessment dilemmas, in Howatson-Jones, L, Standing, M and Roberts, SB (eds) *Patient Assessment and Care Planning in Nursing* (pp94–106). London: Sage/Learning Matters.

Howatson-Jones, L (2012b) Understanding our role in patient assessment, in Howatson-Jones, L, Standing, M and Roberts, SB (eds) *Patient Assessment and Care Planning in Nursing* (pp5–18). London: Sage/Learning Matters.

Hoyle, MT, Alessi, CA, Harker, JO, Josephson, KR, Pietruszka, FM, Koelfgen, M, Mervis, JR, Fitten, LJ and Rubenstein, LZ (1999) Development and testing of a five-item version of the Geriatric Depression Scale. *Journal of the American Geriatrics Society*, 47: 873–8.

International Society of Psychiatric-Mental Health Nurses (ISPN) (2006) *Mission*. Available online at www.ispn-psych.org/html/about_us.html (accessed 13 March 2013).

Johns, C (1996) The benefits of a reflective model in nursing. *Nursing Times*, 92(27): 39–41.

Jones, R (2009) *Mental Health Act Manual* (12th edn). London: Sweet and Maxwell.

Kant, I (1785) *Foundations of the Metaphysics of Morals* (1959 edition). Indianapolis, IN: Bobbs-Merrill Educational Publishing.

Kay, SR, Opler, LA and Lindenmayer, JP (1988) Reliability and validity of the positive and negative syndrome scale for schizophrenics. *Psychiatry Research*, 23: 99–110.

Keaschuk, RA and Newton, AS (2009) The person with an eating disorder, in Barker, PJ (ed.) *Psychiatric and Mental Health Nursing: The craft of caring* (pp278–85). London: Edward Arnold.

Keen, T (2009) Developing collaborative assessment, in Barker, PJ (ed.) *Psychiatric and Mental Health Nursing: The craft of caring* (pp95–104). London: Edward Arnold.

Kennedy, I (2000) *The Inquiry into the Management of Care of Children Receiving Complex Heart Surgery at the Bristol Royal Infirmary*. Bristol: Central Office of Information.

Killick, J and Allan, K (2001) *Communication and the Care of People with Dementia*. Buckingham: Open University Press.

Kitson-Reynolds, E and Rogers, J (2011) Decision making and supervision for third-year student midwives. *British Journal of Midwifery*, 19(2): 125–9.

Kroenke, K and Spitzer, RL (2002) The PHQ-9: a new depression and diagnostic severity measure. *Psychiatric Annals*, 32: 509–21.

Laming, WH (2003) *The Victoria Climbié Inquiry*. Norwich: The Stationery Office.

Laming, WH (2009) *The Protection of Children in England: A progress report*. London: The Stationery Office.

Laurance, J (2003) *Pure Madness: How fear drives the mental health system*. Abingdon: Routledge.

Leape, L, Berwick, D, Clancy, C, Conway, J, Gluck, P, Guest, J, Lawrence, D, Morath, J, O'Leary, D, O'Niell, P, Pinakiewicz, D and Isaac, T (2009) Transforming healthcare: a safety imperative. *Quality & Safety in Healthcare*, 18: 424–8.

Lefebvre, M (2003) Nursing uniforms: dead or alive? *Nursing News*, 7(4), 1–4.

Lorem, GF (2008) Making sense of stories: the use of patient narratives within mental health care research. *Nursing Philosophy: An International Journal for Healthcare Professionals*, 9(1): 62–71.

Lukoff, D, Neuchterlein, KH and Ventura, J (1986) Manual for the expanded Brief Psychiatric Rating Scale (BPRS). *Schizophrenia Bulletin*, 12: 594–602.

Malnutrition Advisory Group (2008) *Malnutrition Universal Screening Tool*. Available online at www.bapen. org.uk/pdfs/must/must_full.pdf (accessed 6 March 2013).

Marieb, EN and Hoehn, K (2010) *Human Anatomy and Physiology* (8th edn). London: Benjamin Cummings.

Mill, JS (1861) *Utilitarianism* (1962 edition). London: Fontana Press.

Mind (2007) *Advocacy in Mental Health*. London: Mind. Available online at www.mind.org.uk/mental_health_ a-z/8040_advocacy_in_mental_health (accessed 10 November 2012).

Mind (2013a) *Clinical Negligence*. Available online at www.mind.org.uk/mental_health_a-z/8048_clinical_negligence (accessed 10 February 2013).

Mind (2013b) *Nearest Relatives under the Mental Health Act*. Available online at www.mind.org.uk/mental_health_a-z/8064_nearest_relatives_under_the_mental_health_act (accessed 27 January 2013).

Morgan, S (2000) *Risk-taking and the 'Risk Business'*. Available online at www.practicebasedevidence.com/files/Risk_Taking_and_the_Risk_Business.pdf (accessed 2 September 2010).

Morgan, S (2007) *Working with Risk Practitioner's/Trainer's Manuals*. Brighton: Pavilion Publishing.

Nash, M (2010) *Physical Health and Wellbeing in Mental Health Nursing*. Maidenhead: Open University Press.

NHS Executive (1993) *A Vision for the Future: The nursing, midwifery and health visiting contribution to healthcare*. London: NHS Executive.

NHS Executive (2000) *Safety, Privacy and Dignity in Mental Health Units: Guidance on mixed sex accommodation for mental health services*. London: Department of Health.

NICE (National Institute for Health and Clinical [now Care] Excellence) (2009) *Depression in Children and Young People: Identification and management in primary, community and secondary care*. London: NICE.

NICE (2011) *Service User Experience in Adult Mental Health: Improving the experience of care for people using adult NHS mental health services* (Clinical Guideline 136, 2011 version). Manchester: NICE. Available online at www.nice.org.uk (accessed 8 March 2013).

NICE (2012) *Service User Experience in Adult Mental Health: Improving the experience of care for people using adult NHS mental health services* (Clinical Guideline 136, 2012 version). London: The British Psychological Society and The Royal College of Psychiatrists. Available online at www.nice.org.uk (accessed 2 April 2013).

NMC (Nursing and Midwifery Council) (2008a) *The Code: Standards of conduct, performance and ethics for nurses and midwives*. London: NMC.

NMC (2008b) *Standards to Support Learning and Assessment in Practice*. London: NMC.

NMC (2009) *Record Keeping: Guidance for nurses and midwives*. London: NMC.

NMC (2010a) *Confirmed Principles to Support a New Framework for Pre-registration Nursing Education*. London: NMC. Available online at www.nmc-uk.org/Get-involved/Consultations/Past-consultations/By-year/Pre-registration-nursing-education-Phase-1-/Confirmed-principles-to-support-a-new-framework-for-pre-registration-nursing-education (accessed 7 March 2013).

NMC (2010b) *Standards for Pre-registration Nursing Education*. London: NMC.

NMC (2011) *Guidance on Professional Conduct for Nursing and Midwifery Students*. London: NMC.

NMC (2012a) *Confidentiality*. Available online at www.nmc-uk.org/Nurses-and-midwives/Advice-by-topic/A/Advice/Confidentiality (accessed 25 January 2013).

NMC (2012b) *Social Networking Sites*. London: NMC. Available online at www.nmc-uk.org/Nurses-and-midwives/Advice-by-topic/A/Advice/Social-networking-sites (accessed 1 April 2013).

Overall, JE and Gorham, DR (1962) The Brief Psychological Rating Scale. *Psychological Reports*, 10: 799–812.

Peplau, HE (1952) *Interpersonal Relations in Nursing: A conceptual frame of reference for psychodynamic nursing*. New York: Putnam.

Peplau, HE (1988 reprint) *Interpersonal Relations in Nursing: A conceptual frame of reference for psychodynamic nursing*. New York: Springer.

Puri, BK, Laking, PJ and Treasaden, IH (2002) *Textbook of Psychiatry* (2nd edn). Edinburgh: Churchill Livingstone.

Rask, M and Brunt, D (2007) Verbal and social interactions in the nurse–patient relationship in forensic psychiatric nursing care: a model and its philosophical and theoretical foundation. *Nursing Inquiry*, 14(2): 169–76.

RCN (Royal College of Nursing) (2009) *Mental Health in Children and Young People: An RCN toolkit for nurses who are not mental health specialists*. London: RCN.

RCN (2013) *Clinical Governance*. Available online at www.rcn.org.uk/development/practice/clinical_governance (accessed 8 April 2013).

Reece, I, Walker, S, Clues, D and Charlton, M (eds) (2006) *Teaching, Training and Learning: A practical guide* (6th edn). Sunderland: Business Education.

Repper, J (2012) Recovery: a journey of discovery, in Tee, S, Brown, J and Carpenter, D (eds) *Handbook of Mental Health Nursing*. London: Hodder Arnold.

Rose, AL and Cheung, M (2012) DSM-5 research: assessing the mental health needs of older adults from diverse ethnic backgrounds. *Journal of Ethnic and Cultural Diversity in Social Work*, 21(2): 144–67.

Rosenberg, W and Donald, A (1995) Evidence based medicine: an approach to clinical problem-solving. *British Medical Journal*, 310: 1122–6.

Ryan, J, Clemmett, S and Perez-Avila, P (1996) Managing patients with deliberate self harm admitted to an accident and emergency observation ward. *Journal of Accident and Emergency Medicine*, 13: 31–3.

Schizophrenia Commission (2012) *The Abandoned Illness: A report from the Schizophrenia Commission*. London: Rethink Mental Illness.

Sharkey, V (2012) Uniform approach. *Nursing Standard*, 26(45): 26–7.

Slade, M, Thornicroft, G, Loftus, L, Phelan, M and Wykes, T (1999) *The Camberwell Assessment of Need (CAN): A comprehensive needs assessment tool for people with severe mental illness*. London: Royal College of Psychiatrists.

Smith, M (2005) Opinion. *Mental Health Practice*, 9(3): 44–5.

Spitzer, RL, Kroenke, K, Williams, JBW and Lowe, B (2006) A brief measure for assessing generalized anxiety disorder. *Archives of Internal Medicine*, 166: 1092–7.

Tham, SW and Ford, TJ (1995) Staff dress on acute psychiatric wards. *Journal of Mental Health*, 4(3): 297–9.

Thompson, C and Dowding, D (2002) *Clinical Decision Making and Judgement in Nursing*. London, Churchill Livingstone.

University of Manchester Centre for Mental Health and Risk (2011) *The National Confidential Inquiry into Suicide and Homicide by People with Mental Illness: Suicide and homicide in Northern Ireland*. Available online at www.medicine.manchester.ac.uk/cmhr/centreforsuicideprevention/nci (accessed 21 February 2012).

Walker, S (2012) Using self-audit to improve nurses' record keeping. *Nursing Times*, 24 August. Available online at www.nursingtimes.net/nursing-practice/clinical-zones/management/using-self-audit-to-improve-nurses-record-keeping/5048667.article (accessed 3 January 2013).

Waterlow, J (2008) *The Waterlow Score*. Available online at www.judy-waterlow.co.uk (accessed 10 April 2013).

Webster, CD, Douglas, KS, Eaves, D and Hart, SD (1997) *HCR–20: Assessing risk for violence* (version 2). Vancouver: Simon Fraser University.

Willis Commission (2012) *Quality with Compassion: The future of nursing education. Report of the Willis Commission on Nursing Education*. London: Royal College of Nursing.

Index